Ludmila Zubkova

Encyclopedia of Clinical and Analytical Dentistry Volume 8

Ludmila Zubkova

Encyclopedia of Clinical and Analytical Dentistry Volume 8

A multi-volume manual

ScienciaScripts

Cover image: www.ingimage.com

This book is a translation from the original published under ISBN 978-620-7-46804-1.

Publisher:
Sciencia Scripts
is a trademark of
Dodo Books Indian Ocean Ltd. and OmniScriptum S.R.L publishing group

120 High Road, East Finchley, London, N2 9ED, United Kingdom
Str. Armeneasca 28/1, office 1, Chisinau MD-2012, Republic of Moldova, Europe
Printed at: see last page
ISBN: 978-620-8-35685-9

Contents

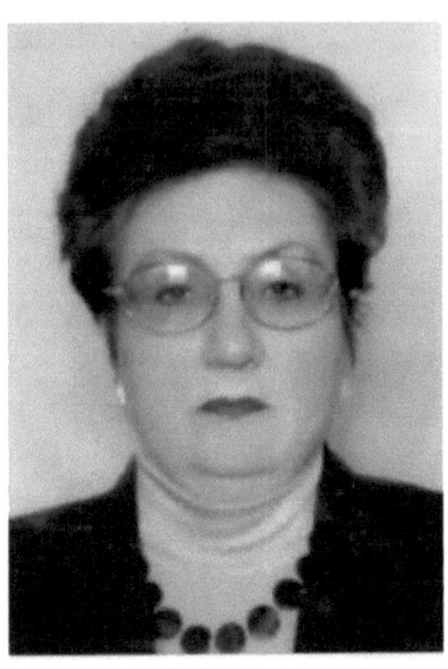

ZUBKOVA LUDMILA PETROVNA
General Director of the Scientific and Clinical Centre "ORTO-DENT" (Odessa, Ukraine
)
"ORTO-DENT (Odessa, Ukraine)
Doctor of Medical Sciences, Professor,
Academician of the Ukrainian Academy of Sciences
EDITOR-IN-CHIEF OF THE MEDICAL INTERNATIONAL JOURNAL
"BIOENERGETICS IN MEDICINE AND BIOLOGY" (Frankfurt, Germany)

CHAPTER 1

Inflammatory-reparative process - non-contagious diseases of the oral **mucosa**

This part (part two) is a continuation of the review of material on the inflammatory-reparative process (IRP) in oral mucosal diseases (OMD), and therefore the numbering of questions (general and private) continues sequentially.

896 (FA-200)	Fundamental aspects	GRP under HIPC
Non-contagious BSORPs are eczematous (general information)?		

In eczema, the "nervous component" is important. Expressed itching, cosmetic defect leads to the development of depression in all patients. The problem of development of such conditions in patients is given considerable attention by doctors of different specialities (including dentists). Electroencephalography (EEG) also belongs to the numerous methods of their diagnostics to a certain extent.

897 (FA-201)	Fundamental aspects	GRP under HIPC
Non-contagious BSORPs are eczematous (EEG and REG values are common)?		

Regarding the diagnostic value of electroencephalogram (EEG) and rheoencephalogram (REEG) parameters in patients,
In particular, in eczema, neurodermatitis, atopic dermatitis, changes in the "brain" electrical potentials (recorded by EEG) and cerebral vascular tone (recorded by REG) were detected, which were non-specific in nature and could be caused by concomitant pathology of the nervous system that occurred in the examined patients. Most often it was recommended to undergo further in-depth examination by neurologists in order to prescribe appropriate therapy (vascular, sedatives, etc.). At the same time, the level of examinations carried out with the help of the above-mentioned methods did not allow drawing conclusions regarding the genesis of the revealed changes depending on the disorders of psychophysiological state of the patients, in particular - and caused by the presence of pronounced itching

of the skin in these allergodermatoses. This did not allow us to recommend the use of specific methods of psychotherapy, including its "training" variants (autotraining, heterotraining, etc.).

898 (FA-202)	Fundamental aspects	GRP under HIPC
Non-contagious BSORPs are eczematous (EEG/REG and histamine/serotonin)?		

An insufficiently solved problem is the question of the relationship between EEG and REG changes and serotonin and histamine metabolism disorders, respectively. These biogenic amines are molecular compounds that can simultaneously fulfil the role of neurotransmitters and mediators of allergy (which is one of the links in the pathogenesis of chronic eczema). It is also known that among the numerous functions of histamine, it also plays the role of an agonist that induces the onset of inflammation, including SORP.

899 (FA-203)	Fundamental aspects	GRP under HIPC
Non-contagious BSORPs are eczematous (EEG/REG and vessels)?		

The vascular system is of paramount importance in this case (as it has already been mentioned many times above), as well as in the past years. Postcapillary venules are the most vulnerable place for the beginning of inflammatory-reparative process development in any organ of the human body.

It is not the "chemoattractant" mechanism of inflammation-reparative process initiation (although it remains one of the most important), but the "cytokine" mechanism that is of primary importance. It is noted that the first cell, which will act on the endothelial cell of the postcapillary venule with its cytokines, should be called a "conductor cell". In the course of autocatalytic process of inflammatory reaction, it attracts other cells, including those that will ensure repair. It is during the inflammatory-reparative process and various mediators (including serotonin and histamine) are "born". However, there is also evidence that changes in serotonin level can influence changes in EEG parameters, and changes in histamine level - in REG. Changes in EEG and REG have also been found in patients with manifestations of depressive states. Thus, there is a need to find out correlations between changes in EEG, REG, psychological research data, serotonin, histamine and their possible significance for the pathogenesis of chronic eczema. Such data can reveal new aspects of development of clinical manifestations of this disease, and, first of all - formation of itching and scratching reflex, development of psychophysiological disorders (up to the degree of depressive states). This is necessary from a practical point of view for the development of new methods of treatment, including non-medication.

900 (FA-204)	Fundamental aspects	GRP under HIPC
Non-contagious BSORP - eczematous (motivational-emotional and autonomic reactions)?		

From the standpoint of modern psychology, holistic behaviour has combined motivational-emotional and autonomic reactions into one functional unit. It is not by chance that the limbic system is defined as both "emotional" and "visceral" brain. If in a healthy person all functions are energetic

In pathology, a pathological psychovegetative state is already formed, within which the relationships between the disturbed motivational-emotional system and the autonomic system are maintained.

inadequate (excessive or insufficient) negative reinforcement.

901 (FA-205)	Fundamental aspects	GRP under HIPC
Non-contagious SARS - eczematous (psycho-vegetative disorders)?		

The degree of psychovegetative disorders well reflects the level of disturbance of adaptive activity, which is provided by the brain and, especially, by the limbic-reticular complex. Psychovegetative disorders are manifested by mental disorders, among which certain phenomena (anxiety, depressive, hypochondriacal, asthenic, hysterical) and vegetative disorders dominate, which are manifested by disorders in many polysystemic shifts. A certain connection of psychovegetative disorders with the character of "brain homeostasis" determined by physiological relationships of activating stem reticular systems with synchronising systems of the brainstem and thalamus has been revealed.

902 (FA-206)	Fundamental aspects	GRP under HIPC
Non-contagious BSORPs are eczematous (brain activation)?		

A. M. Vein et al. concluded that next to psychic and vegetative activations there is also a characteristic brain activation, which is manifested by: 1) a decrease in presentation and amplitude; 2) a tendency to increase the frequency of the main alpha rhythm on the EEG; 3) an increase in its reactivity; and 4) a delayed habituation (fading) of the components of the orientated response. This indicates simultaneous strengthening of activating stem influences both in ascending (decrease of alpha index and other indicated manifestations) and in descending direction - vegetative activation (heart rate, respiration rate, cutaneous-galvanic reflex) and motor activation (clinical and EEG data). All this reflects a holistic ergotropic response, which is characteristic of active goal-directed behaviour, but is distinguished by its inadequacy (out of activity), rigidity and intensity.

903 (FA-207)	Fundamental aspects	GRP under HIPC
Noncontagious BSORPs are eczematous (types of changes in cerebral homeostasis)?		

In recent years, attention has been drawn to the presence of 2 types of changes in brain homeostasis: 1) activating (mentioned above); 2) synchronising. In synchronising changes of brain homeostasis the alpha-index was greater than in activating ones. In this type of changes there are also more intensive psychovegetative disorders and longer duration of the disease. Moreover, descending activation is stored, and ascending - shifts appear to be opposite - that is, synchronisation. The reasons for this situation should be considered: 1) in the light of the concept of so-called "brain tuning": under the influence of prolonged peripheral vegetative activation through afferent brain systems, synchronising shifts occur; 2) it is possible that activation and synchronising shifts are stages in the course of one disease; 3) it is also possible that the "synchronising variant" is based on certain biological regularities, in particular, compensated hypothalamic insufficiency. One way or another, but in such cases there is a violation of physiological relationships between ascending and descending systems of the brainstem reticular forms. Thus, one of the factors in the pathogenesis of autonomic disorders is a disorder of "brain homeostasis", the proper functioning of nonspecific brain systems.

904 (FA-208)	Fundamental aspects	GRP under HIPC
Non-contagious BSORPs are eczematous (sleep-wake biorhythm)?		

It's all about individual patterns psycho-physiological characteristics that are inherent in each of the seven of the states of the sleep-wake cycle:

1) active
2) ordinary
3) relaxed alertness
4) slumber
5) light slow-wave sleep
6) deep, slow sleep
7) REM sleep.

Many patients have a disturbance in the wake-sleep cycle. These are complaints of:

1) asthenic alertness
2) inability to maintain the vigour required for intense activity for long periods of time
3) insomniac disorders
4) less commonly, hypersomnolence.

Objective examination confirms these complaints and mainly reveals increased activation manifestations of sleep:

1) fall asleep longer
2) shortened sleep duration
3) frequent awakenings
4) quantitative and qualitative deficiencies in the slow-wave sleep phase, and especially in deep sleep
5) increased motor activity during sleep.

These disorders come in varying depths and, for example, differ in patients with nocturnal and diurnal crises.

905 (FA-209)	Fundamental aspects	GRP under HIPC
Non-contagious SARS - eczematous (psychovegetative syndrome)?		

Biorhythmological disorders in psychovegetative syndrome are close to those described above: 1) violations of normal circadian oscillations of many autonomic, endocrine and humoral indices are revealed; 2) a picture of desynchronosis is observed; 3) a connection of the occurrence of vegetative paroxysms with the menstrual cycle, season, time of day has been established (evening paroxysms are dominant).

906 (FA-210)	Fundamental aspects	GRP under HIPC
Non-contagious BSORPs are eczematous (meteopathy)?		

In addition to the above-mentioned factors of pathogenesis of autonomic disorders an important place belongs to meteopathy. Meteopathy is an obligatory manifestation of psychovegetative syndrome with crisis course, which occurs in many patients. Meteosensitivity is inherent in many healthy people, and it is possible that they constitute a "risk group" of vegetative disorders. Meteopathy is a manifestation of maladaptation ,
which reflects the functioning of the meteorological system.
non-specific integrative brain systems (EEG).

907 (FA-211)	Fundamental aspects	GRP under HIPC
Non-contagious BSORPs are eczematous (interhemispheric interactions)?		

An important factor in the pathogenesis of vegetovascular suprasegmental disorders may also be a violation of normal interhemispheric interaction.
In patients with neurotic syndromes and vivid psychovegetative disorders smoothing of functional interhemispheric asymmetry is revealed:
1) psychological methods (cerebral dominance index)
2) with EEG examination (compression test)
spectral analysis, EEG mapping).
In pathological states, the representation of individual rhythms and their total power disappear. In fact, there is a shift of the gradient in the opposite direction from the evolutionary path.
This mechanism is thought to reduce adaptive capacity and contribute to the manifestation of psychovegetative syndrome.

908 (FA-212)	Fundamental aspects	GRP under HIPC
Are non-contagious BSORPs eczematous (desegregation)?		

All the above mechanisms (disturbance of brain homeostasis, the role of functional brain states - activity, sleep, biorhythmological aspects, disturbances of interhemispheric interaction) are clearly revealed in psychovegetative syndrome. However, the question is also relevant: are these pathogenetic mechanisms true, or are these processes parallel to psychovegetative dysfunction, and what unites these processes?
With regard to unifying points, it is noted that all cerebral processes are characterised by the fact that they reflect: 1) deficiency of adaptive adaptive functions; 2) disorders of integrative mechanisms of the brain. Psychovegetative disorders are already a reflection of these general disorders, which are defined as "disintegration syndrome".
The marked vivid vegetovascular shifts in paroxysmal states are not in

themselves anti-physiological (rises in blood pressure, increases in heart rate, etc.). But all these vegetovascular shifts become pathological when they occur without connection with normal acts of behaviour. Sympathoadrenal crises that occur outside of active activity or during sleep, parasympathetic shifts that occur in a state of physical tension are reactions that have lost their useful adaptive value and reflect gross violations of adequate vegetative support of activity, the detachment of these vegetative shifts from real behaviour characterise violations of integrative mechanisms of brain activity.

A number of forms of disintegration are considered: intrasystem, intersystem, interhemispheric.

Intrasystem disintegration is manifested by a disruption of physiological relationships between: 1) sympathetic and parasympathetic systems,2) synchronising and
activating apparatuses of the brain. These systems, functioning in reciprocal relations, provide in physiological conditions adequate adaptation to changes in the external and internal environment.

Intrasystemic disintegration is manifested in the disruption of physiological relationships between mental, somatic and motor systems. Such disintegration can be caused by intense itching in chronic eczema (by the mechanism: emotional disturbances - itching - scratching - intensification of emotional disturbances). Psychovegetative activation ceases to be an adequate accompaniment of behaviour, physical and mental activity, and normal psychovegetative relations are disturbed. A model for studying systemic relationships is the "orientated response". In autonomic cerebral pathology, there are not only slowing down of the extinction of its components, but also changes in the order of their
fading, which indicates a disorder of interhemispheric disintegration, the nature of the disturbances of physiological
of interactions between the left and right hemispheres.

Thus, the mechanism of disturbance of the integrative activity of the brain acts as a leading one in suprasegmental vegetovascular disorders and is undoubtedly more complex in comparison with the mechanisms of irritation and destruction (typical for segmental vegetovascular disorders).

909 (FA-213)	Fundamental aspects	GRP under HIPC

Non-contagious BSORPs are eczematous (emotional stress)?

Since the leading factors that cause psychovegetative syndrome are psychic, the role of acute and chronic emotional stress is also obvious. Emotional disorders are the main factor that determines the disruption of normal functioning of non-specific brain systems and causes changes in integrative activity (disintegration syndrome).

910 (FA-214)	Fundamental aspects	GRP under HIPC
Non-contagious BSORPs are eczematous (panic attacks)?		

In recent years, it has been shown the particular importance of right hippocampal insufficiency in panic attacks, i.e.. vegetative paroxysms (to which, to a certain extent, can be attributed and attacks of itching). Often organic and psychiatric factors simultaneously cause the occurrence of psychovegetative syndrome. Important neurochemical features are also studied, such as disorders of lactate-pyruvate metabolism, the provoking role of lactate in some patients in the occurrence of vegetative crises, disorders of glutamate metabolism, insufficiency of brain dopamine systems, the role of latent calcium deficiency; the role of neuropeptide metabolism disorders is also possible.

911 (FA-215)	Fundamental aspects	GRP under HIPC
Non-contagious BSORPs are eczematous (depressions)?		

There is evidence that a decrease in the level of serotonin and noradrenaline and an increase in the expression of receptors for these neurotransmitters is observed in depressive states. If the amount of serotonin and adrenoreceptors increases, against the background of increased levels of norepinephrine - manic syndrome is observed. Lithium reduces the secretion of noradrenaline, the formation of second mediators and increases the expression of adrenoreceptors. It is noted that hyperserotoninaemia is observed in autism, but in 30-50 cases - without visible disorders of serotonin metabolism directly in the brain.

Defects in serotonin transporters are candidates for a root cause of many psychiatric disorders, including depression. It is important to note that some neurons, in particular the Auerbach plexus, synthesise and secrete different neurotransmitters and modulators simultaneously, in particular serotonin, alongside enkephalins and substance P. This may be of significant importance for the development of clinical features of chronic eczema, as there are studies that suggest a triggering role of substance P in relation to itching and a protective role of enkephalins as a response to this sensation.

Thus, the problem of interrelation of disorders in the regulatory structures of the brain, processes of neurotransmitter metabolism (in particular, serotonin and histamine) needs further study and may help to reveal new mechanisms of formation of depressive states in patients with chronic eczema.

912 (FA-216)	Fundamental aspects	GRP under HIPC
Non-contagious BSORPs are eczematous (persistent lesions)?		

The causes of chronicity of HRV (including in eczema) may depend on disorders of the process of "adaptive regeneration" and the development of the process of dysregeneration.

Among numerous factors, this is promoted by changes in reactivity, immune deficiencies, deficiencies of immunocompetent cells and systems of regulation of collagen metabolism, etc. A big role belongs to the disorders of neuroendocrine regulation, insufficiency of vascular and nervous trophics, the presence of hypovitaminosis, suppression of hematopoiesis and other factors.

All this causes a depletion of defence mechanisms, but the volume and duration of the damaging factors matter.

And, despite the specificity of damage, the variety of etiological and pathogenetic mechanisms of disturbance, dysregeneration, as well as adaptive reactions, have fundamentally similar consequences, in which the "breakage" of one of the "links" leads to changes in the whole chain.

In all these cases, due to the disturbance of autoregulatory processes, the links between damage-inflammation-regeneration-repair are "created".

Persistent damage leads to chronic inflammation, and the latter in turn leads to incomplete regeneration.

The above described "vicious circle" closes and a pathological self-sustaining system is formed (which to some extent goes out of the organism's control and sometimes behaves aggressively) - the so-called autocatalytic GRP system.

This "vicious circle" primarily refers to chronic inflammation, which also occurs in eczema and neurodermatitis.

Not only the significant role of IgE-mediated release of histamine from mast cells, but also the non-1dE-mediated release of HRP mediators, especially eicosanoids, may be important in the formed pathological autocatalytic system of HRP in DHF. Prostaglandins and leukotrienes increase vascular permeability and chemoattractant mechanisms to a much greater extent than histamine.

Immunocompetent cells, primarily lymphocytes and antigen-presenting cells, play an important role in eczema.

Their functional activity is largely regulated by cytokines, but in turn, eicosanoids are very important inducers of cytokine synthesis, expression or secretion.

Thus, many cellular systems of both "strictly immune purpose" and "conditionally non-immune purpose" play a role in the development of HRV in eczema and neurodermatitis.

That is why the factors of mast cell degranulation (the main supplier of allergy mediators) can be not only "predominantly immune" molecules (1dE, etc.), but also "conditionally non-immune" (e.g., substance P, eicosanoids), which requires further research both to clarify the pathogenesis of eczema and to improve the methods of treatment of patients.

This also necessitates a comprehensive approach to the therapy of eczema patients with the inclusion of drugs that could influence the processes of formation of relevant molecules at both peripheral and organismal levels.

913 (FA-217)	Fundamental aspects	GRP under HIPC

Non-contagious BSORPs are eczematous (neuropeptide system - common)?

The neuropeptide system (both nociceptive and antinociceptive sections) plays a very important role in ensuring homeostatic processes both at the organism-wide and cellular levels, closely interacting with other molecular regulatory systems.

Neuropeptides, along with other mediators of the nervous system, are specialised in relation to neurons in the brain and spinal cord, but they are also found in other body systems.

To a greater extent, these molecules have an inherent modulating effect because they influence certain mechanisms of functions of various cells that are universal (perception, processing and transmission of information signals) for renewal of the disturbed functional state in one or another system of the organism.

Due to this, neuropeptides regulate both the psychophysiological state of a person (emotions, behaviour, sleep) and the state of many organs and systems, including the digestive system, immune system, adaptation system, etc., through their corresponding receptors (mu-, delta-, kappa-, etc.).

Neuropeptides can provide the necessary effect in much smaller doses than other mediators, and they influence not directly, but indirectly (through other molecular systems) the disturbed mechanisms that lead to pathogenetic changes in a variety of diseases, which is denoted by the term modulation.

914 (FA-218)	Fundamental aspects	GRP under HIPC
Non-contagious BSORPs are eczematous (neuropeptide system - substance P)?		

For example, substance P is contained in the small afferent endings of the posterior horns of the spinal cord. In addition to it, many neurons that terminate in these horns also contain serotonin. When a damaging stimulus excites receptors in the SORP, muscles - there is somatic pain (clearly localised); pain of visceral origin often does not have a clear localisation.

At the same time, both cutaneous and visceral nociceptive sensations, and in SORP lesions, are often accompanied by symptoms of depression and hypochondria.

The genesis of pain in intestinal diseases is often related to impaired motor function, malabsorption syndrome and gas distension of the intestine. In this case, it is particularly important to remember that intestinal cells contain the largest number of opioid receptors.

915 (FA-219)	Fundamental aspects	GRP under HIPC
Non-contagious BSORPs are eczematous (opiate peptides are common)?		

The first step in the manifestation of the biological activity of opiate peptides is their binding to specific receptors on the plasma membrane of target cells, which leads to the formation of a secondary mediator.

For the opiate system, interaction with the receptor usually leads to a decrease in both basal and stimulated concentrations of cAMP, while the long-term effect of opiate peptides causes a long-term decrease in its intracellular concentration. However, over time, the number of adenylate cyclase units gradually increases as a compensatory reaction.

Abrupt opiate withdrawal, while the cell is enriched in adenylate cyclase, abolishes the repression of these units, which in turn leads to a dramatic increase in cAMP concentration and possibly contributes to the development of opiate withdrawal syndrome.

The biosynthesis and secretion of ACTH, beta-endorphin and beta-lipotropic hormone by the pituitary gland are associated with both normal and pathophysiological states of the body.

Immunoreactive beta-endorphin is easily detected and is less susceptible to degradation during storage and processing than ACTH.

916 (FA-220)	Fundamental aspects	GRP under HIPC
Non-contagious BSORPs are eczematous (opiate peptides and pain)?		

Endogenous opiate peptides play a significant role in the regulation of pain impulse transmission. In the posterior horns of the spinal cord, enkephalins are released by interoceptive neurons that interact with afferent pain sensitivity fibres from the periphery. These pain-transmitting fibres form synapses in the grey matter of the posterior horn with another set of neurons; these fibres travel up through the brainstem and cross it to form the lateral spinothalamic pathway. The release of enkephalins (which can be influenced by descending neurons from higher centres) inhibits the release of substance P (a mediator that mediates the transmission of pain impulses) from the afferent fibres that comprise the posterior horn.

917 (FA-221)	Fundamental aspects	GRP under HIPC
Non-contagious BSORPs - eczematous (opiate peptides and other localisations)?		

Endogenous opioid peptides (particularly enkephalins and endorphins) are present not only in the hypothalamus, brain, endocrine glands (pituitary, adrenal glands, ovaries, testes), but also in the GI organs (including the pancreas). These peptides possess:

1) morphine-like analgesic effect
2) by influencing behavioural responses
3) the ability to function as both neurotransmitters and neuromodulators.

This largely determines the role of opioid peptides in the implementation of numerous functions, including memory, stress response, pain impulse transmission, etc., as well as the development of such phenomena as: sedation, irritability, impetuous behaviour. Other phenomena of behavioural disorders (tobacco smoking habit, alcohol use, drug use) may also depend on biochemical disturbances in this system.

918 (FA-222)	Fundamental aspects	GRP under HIPC
Non-contagious BSORPs are eczematous (endorphins and enkephalins are terms)?		

The generalised term "endorphins" is often used, which includes both "enkephalins" (translated as "in the head") and endorphins proper (from the words "endogenous morphine"). However, the molecules of endorphins and enkephalins differ from morphine in their chemical structure, while the molecule of the latter has the property of taking a form similar to that of either enkephalins or endorphins, and such a form can be acquired by the morphine molecule at the moment of its interaction with the corresponding receptors.

Endorphins bind better to opiate receptors than morphine itself, and are 20-700 times stronger than the latter in this respect.

919 (FA-223)	Fundamental aspects	GRP under HIPC
Non-contagious BSORPs are eczematous (endorphins and adaptation system)?		

Taking into account that beta-endorphin (the amount of which is the largest of all endorphins in the organism) and ACTH are derivatives of the same precursor mopecula in the pituitary gland (proopiomelanocortin - POMC), and the synthesis of these two biological compounds is closely related to each other (it is encoded by the same gene), then in case of detecting changes in the level of beta-endorphin it is legitimate to state the presence of changes in ACTH (i.e., not only in the neuropeptide, but also in the adaptive system). That is, the administration of adaptogens necessarily modulates the functional state of the neuropeptide system and, thus, we can consider that from this point of view Echinacea purpurea has a neuropeptide-modulating effect.

At the same time, there are studies that suggest that:

1) differentiated transformation of POMC occurs in different tissues;

2) even in the same organ (e.g. pituitary gland) different POMC derivatives (beta-endorphin, beta-lipotropic hormone, ACTH) are produced in individual cells;

3) in different cells, the end products of POMC secretion are determined by the type of its cleavage by enzyme systems within these cells;

4) Although different cell types may synthesise the same primary gene product, the final profile of hormone secretion may be quite different.

The connection between the neuropeptide system and adaptation systems is also indicated by the fact that enkephalin biosynthesis also occurs in the adrenal glands (in particular, proenkephalin-A, which has 6 repeats of meth-enkephalin and 1 leu-enkephalin sequence in its molecule).

They bind to specific receptors on the plasma membrane of target cells (5 functional types of opioid receptors together with numerous types of endogenous opioids form a complex neuropeptide system), which leads to the formation of secondary mediators (in particular, a long-term decrease in the concentration of cAMP).

The cells that contain endorphin are closely related to the cells in the pancreas that contain insulin. Beta-endorphin stimulates the release of insulin and glucagon, but suppresses the secretion of somatostatin. At the same time, a significant effect of endorphin on carbohydrate metabolism, or any contribution of beta-endorphin to the pathophysiology of SORP has not been established.

Beta-endorphin is present in both the brain and the pituitary gland (and, in the pituitary gland, the cells that contain ACTH and endorphins are in the same locations, and the pituitary gland is thought to have the highest endorphin content in the body).

At the same time, the neurons in which endorphins are biosynthesised are also present in the hypothalamus, they have long branches, and they penetrate into other parts of the brain (in particular, into the limbic system, which is thought to influence memory, learning ability and emotions).

Neurons that contain enkephalins are even more widespread in the CNS, and especially in the posterior spinal cord, an area that contains opiate receptors and conductive pathways involved in the transmission of pain impulses.

Enkephalins are also present in the gastrointestinal tract, and their concentration in the nerve plexus of the intestinal musculature is much higher than in the brain.

Enkephalins are synthesised in the chromophilic cells of the adrenal gland and are stored together with catecholamines in the same secretory granules. Enkephalin release occurs as part of the sympathetic stress response along with the release of adrenaline and noradrenaline.

The release of enkephalins (which can be influenced by descending neurons from upstream centres) inhibits the release of substance P (i.e. the mediator that mediates the transmission of pain impulses) from afferent fibres that are part of the posterior horn of the spinal cord.

Evidence is presented that administration of opioid peptides to animals at doses lower than those required to achieve analgesia leads to the development of specific and vulnerable behavioural reactions (such as severe seizures, stereotyped behaviours, and even superaggression).

Endorphins play a role in appetite regulation and may be responsible for eating disorders. The site of action of endorphin that affects appetite is the paraventricular nucleus of the hypothalamus. Taking into account what has been said above (the presence of opiate receptors in the GI tract, the synthesis of beta-endorphin in the pancreas, where it stimulates insulin release, which leads to a change in glucose utilisation), we can state the need to influence the neuropeptide system by normalising the functioning of the GI tract.

From the point of view of immunorehabilitation, the most recognised are preparations of Echinacea, Eleutherococcus, Ginseng, Rhodiola rosea, and Aralia manchuriana, which are largely adaptogens, but also affect the immunity system and the activity of immune reactions.

920 (FA-224)	Fundamental aspects	GRP under HIPC
Non-contagious BSORP - eczematous (adaptogens - echinacea)?		

At the same time, in recent years it has been emphasised that preparations of Echinacea purpurea belong not only to adaptogens, but also to immunotropic preparations of plant origin with a pronounced immunomodulatory property, which depends on its constituents.

Echinacea is a perennial herbaceous plant of the aster family, all parts of which contain polysaccharides and essential oil (flowers - 0.5 %, herb - up to 0.35 %, roots - from 0.05-0.25 %). The main constituent of the essential oil is non-cyclic sesquiterpenes. In the roots found glycoside echinacoside, resins, organic acids (palm-itinic, linoleic, cerotinic), as well as - phytosterols. The main active substance, which has immunostimulating activity, are polysaccharides of Echinacea.

921 (FA-225)	Fundamental aspects	GRP under HIPC
Non-contagious BSORP - eczematous (echinacea - mechanisms of action)?		

Echinacea purpurea exerts its immunocorregulatory effect due to the content of important trace elements (selenium, zinc, etc.), biologically active substances (betaine, rutin, flavone glycosides, enzymes, etc.), vitamins (A, C). This complex of substances, which is included in the composition of Echinacea purpurea, provides such mechanisms of action.

1. Stimulates cellular and humoral reactions of nonspecific immunity, i.e. it has immunomodulatory effect in different ways: strengthening of antibody synthesis; activation of phagocytosis (by neutrophils and macrophages); influence on the functions of macrophages (bactericidal, cytotoxic, secretion of interferon, TNF, IL-1); stimulates chemotaxis of granulocytes; stimulates transformation of B-lymphocytes into plasma cells; improves the functions of T-helpers.
2. In addition, Echinacea purpurea has and anti-inflammatory effect, which is due to: inhibition of cyclooxygenase or 5-lipoxygenase (ie, prevents the increased formation of prostaglandins and leukotrienes); by stimulating the adrenal cortex and increasing the synthesis of endogenous glucocorticoids.
3. With prolonged use - increases non-specific resistance of the body to unfavourable environmental factors (is a biogenic stimulator of the CNS, adaptogen).
4. Carries out bacteriostatic, antiviral and antimycotic action (inhibits the growth and reproduction of streptococcus, staphylococcus, Escherichia coli, influenza viruses, herpes).
5. It has an analgesic effect on burns.

922 (FA-226)	Fundamental aspects	GRP under HIPC
Non-contagious BSORPs are eczematous (echinacea - application)?		

Due to the above properties, Echinacea purpurea is used as part of complex therapy for many chronic diseases.

diseases (respiratory diseases, peptic ulcer disease, arthritis, hepatitis, nephritis and dental diseases), infectious diseases (viral, septic, infected wounds and burns), pathological conditions in case of weakening of the immune system (caused by chronicisation of inflammatory diseases, in case of weakened immune system (caused by chronic inflammatory diseases, influence of ionising radiation, UVB, chemotherapeutic drugs, long-term antibiotic therapy), metabolic disorders (diabetes mellitus, liver diseases), action of various chemical substances of toxic nature, which are contained in the air and foodstuffs (heavy metals, pesticides, insecticides, fungicides), etc.).

923 (FA-227)	Fundamental aspects	GRP under HIPC
Non-contagious BSORP - eczematous (echinacea - indications are common)?		

According to the division of immunotropic therapy into immunostimulatory, immunosuppressive , and immunomodulatory, in accordance with the peculiarities of eczema and neurodermatitis development in children, in our opinion, the latter should be used to the greatest extent, which is aimed at restoring the immune status to a balanced state and is often used in persons with the presence of manifestations of psychoemotional disorders, increased fatigue syndrome, as well as - in severe patients who are at risk of developing immunodeficiency or autoimmune process.

It should also be taken into account that the mechanisms of IgE-independent degranulation of basophils involve complement products, chemokines, substance P and others. In case of action of the above mentioned damaging factors, mechanisms of activation of membrane phospholipids of basophils/touch cells are switched on, and stages with a number of effects occur, which testify to activation of both types of basophils. This promotes changes in the functional state of other cells as well, including the mediators we have studied :

monocytes/macrophages - leukotriene B4; neutrophils - leukotriene B4; basophils/mast cells - prostaglandins. Given that receptors to opioid peptides have been identified on immunocompetent cells (in particular, on lymphocytes), inflammatory mediators (eicosanoids) may also cause a feedback response from the neuropeptide system.

In addition, mast cells are also abundant in the GI tract organs, and the increased release of prostaglandins and leukotrienes from them leads to a reaction from the vascular and muscular systems of these organs with clinical manifestations of irritation (symptoms of discomfort, pain).

That is, a peculiar "vicious circle" of pathophysiological changes in children with eczema and neurodermatitis is formed at the level of GI organs, involving markers of nociception (substance P), antinociception (beta-endorphin, meth-enkephalin, leu-enkephalin), inflammation (PGE2, PGF2-alpha, leukotriene B4).

Thus, the use of general physiological principles of functioning, so to speak, of a unified "neuroendocrine-immune system" - the principle of the "neuroendocrine-immune system" - becomes important.
sensitivity of feedback receptors as the leading mechanism responsible for the character of oscillations of the corresponding regulatory molecular systems of cell populations. In this case, it is promising to use drugs that, even when administered topically, can simultaneously act on both the neuropeptide system and the eicosanoid system. This treatment may become more effective when drugs that affect both immunocompetent cells (preferably with a mild immunomodulatory effect) and drugs that are able to block the entry of allergens through one of the main routes of their entry into the body - the GI tract (for example, sorbents, and those that are available for widespread implementation in practice and the doctor has sufficient experience in their use) are used in the system of general therapy.

924 (FA-228)	Fundamental aspects	GRP under HIPC
Non-contagious SIBRS - psoriasis, red squamous lichen planus (overview)?		

These two nosological forms are usually brought to one lecture, seminar or practical training. Meanwhile, it is known that in spite of certain identical points (primary element of the rash - papule, presence of Kebner's phenomenon, unknown etiological factor, etc.) - these are independent diseases, the pathogenesis of which is significantly different, and many aspects of them need further study; psoriasis often affects SORP (in the expanded form of "haematological" and "oncological" topics), the subject of future volumes of the encyclopaedia, but some of its sections are relevant to the problem of GRP.

925 (FA-229)	Fundamental aspects	GRP under HIPC
Non-contagious BSORP - psoriasis (assumption #1)?		

The problem of psoriasis, from the earliest times (labelled as "the devil's rose") to the present day, has been, and still is, unresolved in the most essential points, and - Auspitz's question "Was psoriasis ist?" ("What is psoriasis?") has not received a definitive answer.

In this encyclopaedia, we do not aim at a comprehensive coverage of the problem of psoriasis, but will focus only on some aspects of the development of inflammatory-reparative process in this disease.

But before turning to aspects of the inflammatory-reparative process in psoriasis, in view of the fact that one of the distinctions of this encyclopaedia is the consideration not only of factual material but also of - hypotheses or concepts, we ~ 35 ~ will review the assumptions and certain lines of enquiry for the solution of the problem.

First assumption. It is possible that in the direct meaning ("etiological factor") no "virus" (in the microbiological interpretation of this word) will be found, and the "virus" may be a "failure" in the cellular programme(s) - so to speak in the "computer interpretation of the concept of virus".

926 (FA-230)	Fundamental aspects	GRP under HIPC
Non-contagious BSORP - psoriasis (assumption #2 - "DNIES")?		

The second assumption. It is closely connected with the first one. Even biochemical and cytological studies of the past years proved that "in response to any damage of any cellular compartments, ALL its molecular systems take part, to a greater or lesser extent," which we have pointed out earlier.

Modern research has proven the existence of a single neuroendocrine-immune regulatory system in the body, or as it is more commonly referred to DNIES - Diffuse NeuroImmunoEndocrine System. Cell signalling occurs according to general principles, and hormonal regulation is a GENERAL biologic phenomenon that is inherent to any cell, regardless of its origin and basic biological role in the organism. The term "hormone" now refers to a variety of signalling molecules and many of them have already been classified (e.g. eicosanoids, cytokines, etc.). Consideration of already known molecules in terms of their functioning and ensuring the actions of the diffuse neuroimmunoendocrine system has already allowed many medical specialties to carry out research at finer levels of the organisation of cells and subcellular organelles and to obtain additional evidence of the existence of a common chemical language of intercellular communication in the nervous, immune and endocrine systems. There is no doubt that hormonal function is not a specific activity of individual cells, but has a general biological significance and is inherent in any living cell, regardless of their origin and main role in the organism.

Further development of integral views on molecular cellular (intercellular) processes will at least allow to expand the knowledge of many pathological processes in dentistry.

927 (FA-231)	Fundamental aspects	GRP under HIPC
Non-contagious BSORP - psoriasis (assumption #3 - immunogenetics)?		

The third assumption. It is also closely related to the previously discussed fundamental aspects of SORP . It is possible that failures with the study of etiopathogenesis of psoriasis depend on the fact that we are "accustomed" to a certain interpretation of some terms, and given that the formation of a new basic integral field of knowledge of neuroimmunoendocrinology has only just begun, we are "not ready" to make unexpected interpretations of traditional views. One of the promising directions may be the revision of our attitude to the problem of "ANTIGEN" in general. Most often under this concept in textbooks and in scientific literature they mean "Alien". But it is not exactly and not always so, as we interpret it literally.

It is not by chance that geneticists believe that "non-genetic diseases do not exist". This does not mean that all of them are hereditary, but the fact that nothing happens in the cell without genes is a truth (although not always proven). In relation to the majority of antigens (T-dependent), no immune response takes place without the participation of genes of the major histocompatibility complex (HLA in humans).

Indeed, most foreign molecules

is captured by antigen-presenting cells, in which "processing" takes place, during which fragments of the foreign molecule are combined with HLA genes and displayed on the surface of APCs in the complex "fragment of foreign molecule + HLA", which is the actual antigenome. The T-helper recognises the HLA genes of APCs (therefore, the term "antigen" should be logically abbreviated not as Ag or AG, but as AG); considering that they are "contaminated", the foreign molecule sends a "help" signal to B cells; the same signal "helps" the B cell to transform into a plasma cell with the output to the "protection command" of the humoral immune response molecules (antibodies-immunoglobulins).

To date, HLA genes have already been investigated in SORP diseases and there are initial results, and this problem is promising for further study.

928 (FA-232)	Fundamental aspects	GRP under HIPC
Non-contagious BSORP - psoriasis (assumption #4 - immuno-oncology)?		

Fourth assumption . If we are talking about the integration of research, then, in our opinion, promising in the study of psoriasis is the use of experience regarding tumour antigens, which are carried out in oncology (which even made it possible to create a separate direction in the treatment of cancer patients - ADOPTIVE therapy).

Thus, one of the modern approaches to solving the problem of pathogenesis of chronic diseases is to determine the levels of markers of certain processes in the organism (cancer, inflammation, etc.).

The term "marker" is broadly defined as a characteristic property, a label, a mark, a specific feature.

Given the environmental stress in many regions of the world, the problem of identifying both cancer markers and biomarkers in the broader sense of the term is of particular importance in dental practice.

In most cases, each cell type (or cell type phenotypes) expresses specific polypeptides, and the identification of these specific features is widely used for disease diagnosis (chromosomal, immune, tumour, enzyme markers, etc.).

There is evidence for specific use of markers in SORP lesions/diseases as well.

Thus, it is noted that:

1) The chromosomal marker of T-cell lymphoma is transposition (a type of chromosomal abnormality - 7, 14 or 11 or 9) with possible oncogenes tel-

1, tel-2, tel-3;

2) HA markers (expression of alloantigens (aG) of the major histocompatibility complex) can be used to diagnose dermatitis herpetiformis (aG-Dw3), psoriasis vulgaris (aG-Cw6), vesicular vulgaris (aG-DR4 and aG-A10), as well as reactive arthritis of gonorrhoeal etiology (aG-B27), psoriatic arthritis (aG-Bw38).

At the same time, the above-mentioned chromosomal markers indicate only a relative risk of the development or existence of the respective disease (from 4.8 to 18.0 per cent)

The so-called "**oncomarkers**" are much more reliable in terms of diagnostic value: CA-125 (ovarian cancer), CA-15-3 (metastatic breast cancer), prostate-AG (prostate cancer).

929 (FA-233)	Fundamental aspects	GRP under HIPC
Non-contagious BSORP - psoriasis (CD markers; clusters)?		

CD markers (CD-aG; clusters of differentiation) have been widely used in immunodiagnosis.

Different clusters (accumulation and/or association of previously unconnected homogeneous cells, molecules, etc.) appear on lymphocytes at different stages of their differentiation:

1) AG-independent differentiation of lymphocytes takes place in the thymus (**lymphocytes** of the thymus are called **thymocytes** for this reason);

2) Stage 1:

a) T-lymphocyte progenitor cell enters the thymus from the bone marrow in the foetal period and can express differentiated AG -CD7 on its surface;

б) this cell then synthesises the cytoplasmic form of the C molecule D3;

в) then it exposes on its surface C D1 and CD2;

Stage 2: protimocyte

a) already has a CD7 phenotype$^+$, CD1$^+$, CD2$^+$, c CD3$^+$, CD4$^-$, 0)8;

б) CD molecule disappears when the cell matures and the cytoplasmic form of C D3+ (with CD3) moves into the membrane;

в) stage: thymocyte - in the process of assembly of a- and b-chains of the Tlim phocyte prothymocyte receptor:

а) begin to express CD4 and CD markers, giving rise to the majority of thymocytes with CD1+, CD2+, CD3+, CD4+ phenotype$^-$, CD8 ;$^+$

б) these cells are capable of differentiating in two directions:

- into CD1 cells$^+$, CD2$^+$, CD4$^+$, CD8 ;$^-$
- into CD1$^+$, CD2$^+$, CD4$^-$, CD8+ cells;
- in the presence of the membrane marker CD3 and T-lymphocyte av receptor in both subtypes;

в) these cells are already "allowed" to leave the thymus, they appear in the peripheral blood and lymphoid organs and are normally detached from the thymus ;

T lymphocytes express either CD4 or CD8, and cells of CD4+, CD8+ phenotype are absent.

In the cortical layer of the thymus, maturing T-lymphocytes are protected from the action of Ig from the internal environment of the organism due to the haematotic barrier existing here (it is formed by endothelial cells, basal membrane of capillaries of the cortical layer, perivascular connective tissue and its cells (pericytes and macrophages), dendritic epithelial cells with their membrane).

Thymocytes from the cortical layer enter the cerebral layer, where they differentiate into C D4+ and CD8+ lymphocytes.

Mature T-lymphocytes leave the brain layer through venules and lymphatic vessels (only 3-5%). The last cells die (they are neutralised by macrophages present here).

930 (FA-234)	Fundamental aspects	GRP under HIPC
Non-contagious BSORP - psoriasis (molecular markers; monoclonal antibodies)?		

The use of immunocytochemical methods makes it possible to establish the localisation of both molecular structures and molecular compounds - Ig, hormones, enzymes, AG, receptors. Modern improvements in methodological techniques (direct and indirect immunoenzyme, cytochemical methods, reactions using unlabelled antibody (aT)-enzyme complexes and highly sensitive systems for visualisation of binding sites of unlabelled aT to aG, creation of hybrid technology for production of monoclonal aT, etc.) have contributed to significant advances in the

diagnosis of leukaemia and tumours, and to the specification of relevant molecular markers.
The use of immunocytochemical methods provides valuable information:
1) on the origin of leukaemic cells;
2) the histogenesis of various neoplasms (which is important for the choice of rational treatment regimens);
3) marker immunocytochemical reactions allow to establish the cellular nature of metastases, especially in case of unclear localisation of the primary tumour, as well as to detect micrometastases in lymph nodes, bone marrow, in exudates from serous cavities;
4) obtaining monoclonal AT to a wide range of lineage-specific, differentiated and activating AT- and B-lymphocytes, granulocytes, erythroblastic cells and SMF allowed to unite numerous leukocytic AGs into 247 differentiation clusters; it also facilitated immunophenotyping of lymphoid forms of leukaemia and non-Hodgkin's malignant lymphoma;
5) in immunohistochemical diagnostics of solitary tumours, a wide arsenal of mono- and polyclonal AT to tissue- and organ-specific AGs, hormones, enzymes and products of oncogenes is used in the study of histological sections and thin-needle biopsies; this became possible due to detailed study of the structure, synthesis and expression of marker AGs (expression is stored in cells and in the process of their malignant transformation).
At the present stage in haematology, the diagnosis of haemoblastosis is carried out comprehensively, in accordance with the classification of diseases (analysis of signs: morphological + immunophenotypic + molecular-genetic + clinical; this, for example, allowed:
1) to identify prognostically significant disease variants (by immunophenotyping using an appropriate panel of monoclonal aTs);
2) Determine markers for certain haematoblastosis processes, e.g:
- megakaryocytic differentiation (expression of CD41, CD42, CD61);
- minimal signs of differentiation in acute myeloid leukaemia (expression of at least one of the panmyeloid AGs: CD33, GD13, GD117);
3) To better characterise the nature of cells in chronic lymphoproliferative diseases.

931 (FA-235)	Fundamental aspects	GRP under HIPC

Non-contagious BSORP - psoriasis (cancer markers)?

In oncology, the choice of markers that allow the identification of the main types of neoplasms (epithelial, connective tissue, lymphoid, melanoma, etc.) and diagnose tumour metastases (including micrometastases), detect even isolated tumour cells (Tg-se1k). Such markers include low molecular density cytokeratins (GD45), melanoma-associated AG (NMV-45) and others. Cytokeratins are found in the majority of low-differentiated cancer tumours.

Certain peculiarities of formation of known tumour antigens have been noted. However, despite the advances in tumour diagnosis using oncomarkers, the problem of searching for new possibilities of "marker" research remains unsolved.

Attention is paid to molecular and genetic mechanisms of neoplastic cells origin and life activity, progression of oncopathology under the influence of carcinogenic factors, links between the development of neoplastic processes and changes at a certain level (oncogenes, oncosuppressor and mutator genes). Data have been obtained that one of the manifestations of genetic propensity to oncopathology is the phenomenon of primary-multiple localisation of the neoplastic process.

932 (FA-236)	Fundamental aspects	GRP under HIPC
Non-contagious BSORP - psoriasis (cancir ogeni)?		

Attention is drawn to the following:

1) According to the Convention No. 139 on Occupational Cancer (Geneva, 1974), persons who are exposed to carcinogenic factors at work must be notified of this, which is also supported by the relevant Ukrainian state regulation (Order No. 25 of 07.02.1997, "List of substances ... carcinogenic for humans" with additions of 2006);

2) It is necessary to pay attention during medical examinations to so-called pre-cancerous conditions, and it is advisable to use known laboratory markers of cancer risk when forming risk groups (in our

opinion, to a certain extent, such markers can include elemental examination);

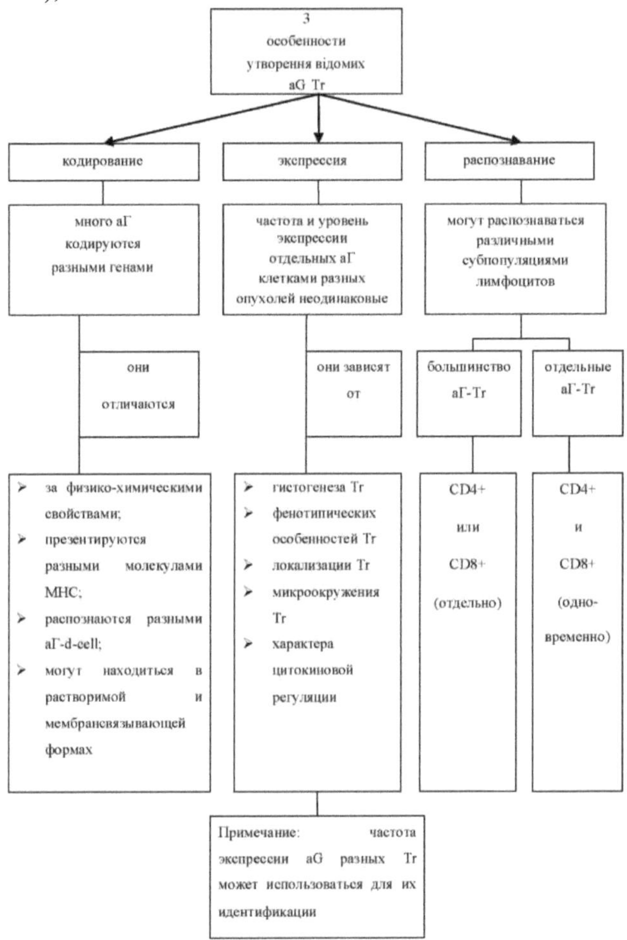

Fig. Some mechanisms of tumour (Tr) antigen (aG) formation

3) a wide variety of factors can lead to the modification of normal cells into cancer, resulting in a reorientation of enzymatic systems without gross changes in protein structure, immunological specificity, and the like.

933 (FA-237)	Fundamental aspects	GRP under HIPC
Non-contagious BSORPs - psoriasis (oncoimmunology referrals)?		

Having analysed the state of research in modern oncoimmunology, 7 main directions are distinguished.

The highlighted main directions of oncoimmunology may be relevant to the problem of psoriasis as well. These directions are as follows:

1) identification of tumour-associated AGs (tumour-associated specific - products of mutant genes);

2) studying the patterns of tumour peptide recognition by aG-recognizing cells (aG -d-sep - antigen-recognizing (diagnostic) cells) in parallel with the study of intracellular mechanisms of the process of presentation of a G-antigen-presenting (present) cells (aG p-sc11);

3) studies of mechanisms of realisation of cytotoxic action of different effector cells (E f-sel);

4) studies of the peculiarities of cytokine regulation of immune system cells (Im-cell); the influence of cytokines on tumour cells and their interaction with immune system cells;

5) elucidation of mechanisms of tumours "slipping" from immunological control, factors of immunostimulation of tumour growth and their suppressive effect on immune system cells;

6) search for informative methods of immunological studies as criteria for assessing the condition of cancer patients and the effectiveness of immunotherapy;

7) development of new approaches to immunotherapy of patients with malignant tumours based on the results of fundamental research.

934 (FA-238)	Fundamental aspects	GRP under HIPC
Non-contagious BSORP - psoriasis (identification of aH)?		

Currently, entire groups of both Tr-specific and non-specific aGs (MAGE, BAGE, GAGE, NY-ESO, LAGE, PAGE, MART, more than 30 melanoma aGs, etc.), including genes encoding them, have already been identified. Given the importance of the processes of aG-Tg recognition and immune response induction, anti-Tg therapies targeting these mechanisms are being developed.

It is advisable to use so-called radio-protective nutrition.

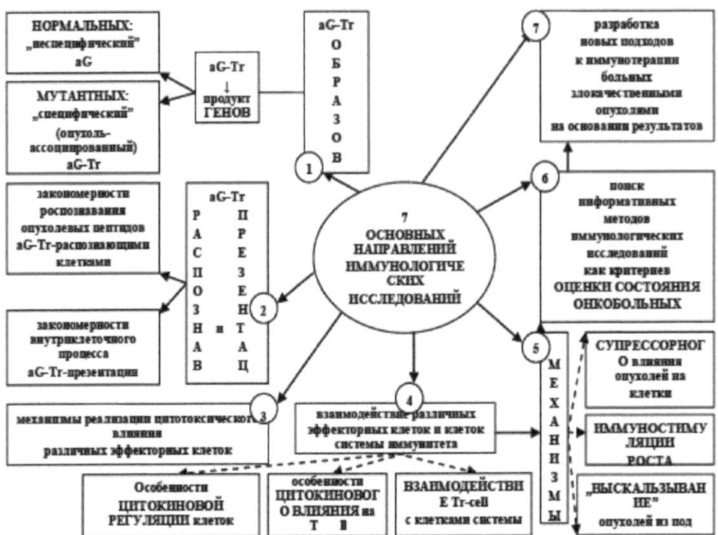

Fig. Main directions of immunological research in oncology that can be used in dentistry

The identification of aG (aG) has numerous difficulties, among which the main ones are also at least 7 that are related to the viability of Tg-se11 :

1) expression of aG-Tg-se11 is either absent or negligible;
2) aG secretion by many Tg-se11 is weak (they are absent both in blood and in body fluids);
3) the presence of various AG-determinant epitopes in Tg-cells (including those inherent to normal cells);
4) Instability of the Tg-se11 AG structure at different stages of tumour growth;
5) Difference in the aG -structure of primary and metastasising Tg ;
6) not all AGs are capable of inducing antitumour defence;
7) some AGs can cause stimulation of Tg growth.

935 (FA-239)	Fundamental aspects	GRP under HIPC
Non-contagious BSORP - psoriasis (promising directions)?		

The following are promising in this respect referrals as getting information to start treatment:

1) on the presence of conditions necessary for the process of aG-Tg recognition (first of all, which aG -Tg and MNS are expressed by this or that Tg-se11);
2) about Tg peptides that induce anti-tumour defences;
3) about peptides that contribute to "slipping" Tg from recognition.
Unjustified use of one or another aG for vaccination may be a factor in the ineffectiveness of certain vaccine therapies. Previous testing of Tg-se11 is necessary to obtain information about its phenotypic features that are important for the induction of tumour response (i.e., control not only at the cellular level but also at the molecular level, including the genome).

936 (FA-240)	Fundamental aspects	GRP under HIPC
Non-contagious BSORP - psoriasis (aH expression)?		

Recognition of AGs of any nature occurs only when the target cell and lymphocytesexpress identical MNS AGs.
It is this strict regularity that explains the fundamental position that the study of the processes of AG-Tg recognition is in direct connection with the study of MNS AG expression in both Tg-se11 and lymphocytes. At present, the role of MNS aG expression has been clarified:
1) The frequency of expression of class I and class II MNS AGs is different in cells of different tumours;
2) expression of class I MNS AGs is reduced already at the stage of pre-tumour states;
3) In a number of cases, there is a "negative" correlation between the expression of class I MNS AG and T progression in many tumours: intestinal, breast, cervical, oral cavity and larynx, and bladder;
4) a dramatic decrease in class I MNS AG expression coincides with early metastasis, which is especially true for melanoma cells, which are generally characterised by deficient class I MNS AG expression and poor immunogenicity;
5) The intensity of the reduction in the expression of class I MNS AGs varies depending on the localisation of Tg and the baseline expression level of these AGs .

937 (FA-241)	Fundamental aspects	GRP under HIPC
Non-contagious BSORP - psoriasis (assumption #5)?		

Fifth assumption. The mechanisms of known "phenomena" cannot be considered to have been definitively elucidated; this also applies to the mechanism(s) for the development of the Kebner phenomenon (isomorphic reaction).

This phenomenon occurs not only in psoriasis, but also in other diseases (red flat lice, vitiligo, etc.). It is possible that some features of the rash in other diseases ("along the course of nerves", there is even a suggestion that the rash may be localised "along the course of acupuncture meridians", etc.) also occur according to the "scenario" of Kebner's phenomenon.

The inflammatory process that develops in Kebner's phenomenon resembles a hypersensitivity reaction.

Another problem is that sometimes doctors sometimes make mistakes in diagnosing Kebner's phenomenon and may mistake it for, for example, herpes zoster.

At the same time, the presence of Kebner's phenomenon indicates the progressive stage of the disease and necessitates a differentiated approach to the choice of therapy.

938 (FA-242)	Fundamental aspects	GRP under HIPC
Non-contagious BSORP - psoriasis (readiness for hyperplasia)?		

According to many scientists, psoriasis also essentially resembles a neoplastic process, because in this dermatosis the main phenomenon is "unrestrained mitosis of keratinocytes". But, as in tumours, the existence of the psoriatic antigen (a G) is considered doubtful by many authors.

Since T-cell activation has been detected in psoriatic plaques, it is assumed that it is caused by antigenic determinants that appear in the event of cell destruction (e.g., mechanical - Koebner reaction; localisation of the rash in

the area of the most traumatised sites).
Thus, the study of the essence of the Kebner reaction in psoriasis and red squamous plaque remains an urgent problem and requires detailed study both in pathophysiological and
practical aspects.
However, the analysis of modern literature, which partially covers this problem, gives grounds to consider from other positions the role of both these damaging factors in the mechanisms of development of pathophysiological changes in Kebner's phenomenon in psoriasis patients and the already known ones.
This is especially true when considering the problem of the recently discovered adaptation-trophic function of the autonomic nervous system (its third division found in the intestine and the role of the so-called "trophogens").
The trigger factor can be any external or internal stimulus, and under its influence in the process of adaptation, the regulatory circuit that controls mitosis and their synthesis of keratin, lipids and other biologically active substances is disrupted.
In the process of interaction, the activity of individual coenzymes may change, which in general leads to disorganisation of biochemical cycles.
At the final stage there occurs: on the one hand - 1) decrease of keylon formation; 2) decrease of sensitivity of keratinocyte receptors to the action of : a) adrenaline - keylon complex, b) decreased formation of cAMP; on the other hand - 3-a) increased formation of aldosterone; 3-b) increased concentration of epidermal growth factor, which, in turn, leads to a violation of the intracellular ratio of sodium and potassium ions, increased secretion of histamine and other biologically active substances, violation of the ratio of cAMP/ cGMP .

939 (FA-243)	Fundamental aspects	GRP under HIPC
Non-contagious BSORPs - psoriasis (role of cAMP/ cGMP relationship)?		

The level of cell division in psoriasis is known to be 1000 times greater than in normal psoriasis. The rate of division is controlled to a large extent by the balance between cAMP and cGMP An increase in cAMP levels is usually associated with decreased proliferation, while an increase in cGMP is associated with increased cell proliferation. In the skin and POPR of psoriasis patients, higher levels of cGMP and reduced levels of cAMP are observed. Thus, cAMP inhibitors create conditions for increased (excessive) proliferation. Stimulators of cGMP also lead to the same.

The disturbance of the relationship between cyclic nucleotides (decrease in cAMP and increase in cGMP) directly depends on their regulating enzymes (adenylate cyclase and phosphodiesterase). One of the factors of such a disturbance of cyclic nucleotide relationships may be an increase in the level of eicosanoids.

It should be noted that the overwhelming majority of studies on cyclic nucleotides concern their content in one or another medium of the organism. Certainly, absolute extrapolation of the data obtained with respect to the content of substances in SORP and blood is not sufficiently reliable, but at the same time, one cannot ignore the facts that: first, through special regulatory mechanisms, cyclic nucleotides can sharply increase the activity of phosphodiesterases, and then their content in the cell will decrease; second, in many types of cells, it can be observed that prolonged stimulation of adenylate cyclase leads to a 3-phase change in the concentration of cAMP:

the increase in concentration is modified by a plateau and then a decrease to the initial level.

This may be due to the fact that the substance that activates adenylate cyclase, indirectly, through an increase in the concentration of cAMP, increases the activity of phosphodiesterase; thirdly, we cannot ignore the levels of these biologically active substances in the blood, because they are non-specific markers of inflammation and other pathological processes, and their study in the dynamics of treatment can be considered as a criterion of its effectiveness.

940 (FA-244)	Fundamental aspects	GRP under HIPC
Non-contagious BSORPs - psoriasis (role of axon-reflex)?		

It is possible that the Kebner phenomenon is a reaction that develops according to the "script" of a reflex (axon-reflex is a reflex reaction that is carried out, unlike a true reflex, without the involvement of central nervous mechanisms).

In the axon-reflex, the excitation which originates in a peripheral nerve ending, TRANSFERS TO THE POINT OF DEVELOPMENT of a centrifugal fibre from one branch to another, Causing a definite physiological effect.

Eicosanoids occupy a significant place, but it is possible that nucleotides are also involved. This requires the prescription of drugs that would affect the levels of these bioactive compounds in psoriasis patients.

941 (FA-245)	Fundamental aspects	GRP under HIPC
Non-contagious BSORP - psoriasis (readiness to develop GDM)?		

The abnormalities in eicosanoids, second cell mediators, and neurotransmitters detected in psoriasis patients may indicate not only the "readiness" of patients to develop inflammation (including the mechanism of the Kebner phenomenon), but also the "readiness" of the nervous system, which is unable to influence the prevention of inflammation development (by the axon-reflex mechanism). Consequently, in addition to the relatively well-studied functions of the autonomic nervous system (sympathetic and parasympathetic influences), disorders are also observed in such a function as adaptation and trophic. Thus, the data obtained in the past years about numerous disorders of various systems of the organism need to be revised, taking into account the essence and importance of this function. It is not excluded that the development of isomorphic reaction is also possible

(Kebner's phenomenon) is also largely dependent on disorders in the structural components of the autonomic nervous system.

942 (FA-246)	Fundamental aspects	GRP under HIPC
Non-contagious BSORP - psoriasis (treatment with phytoniringa preparations)?		

In the system of complex treatment of psoriasis patients use preparations created according to the principles of phytoniring (from English phyton - plant and engineering - engineering), for example - from willow bark (asalix, etc.) - refers, in fact, to the means that are called "prodrugs", because the active substances of this drug are in the form of a prodrug mixture, which does not have an irritating effect on the gastrointestinal tract.

The main advantage of this drug is that it simultaneously inhibits lipoxygenase, hyaluronidase and formation of free radicals, and not only is not inferior in efficiency to COX-2 inhibitors, but at some points is much stronger and much cheaper.

Randomised, double-blind, placebo-controlled studies have been carried out in relation to its efficacy in different diseases. These effects of Assalix depend not only on salicin, but also on other components that also have the ability to inhibit lipoxygenase, hyaluronidase and free radical formation (the "cumulative effect" of flavonoids, tannins, salicylates and other constituents).

Assalix in the system of complex treatment of patients with psoriasis has a pronounced anti-inflammatory effect (restoration to physiological values of most of the studied parameters).

Taking into account that in the presence of Kebner's phenomenon it restores almost to physiological values the ratios of cAMP/ cGMP and (to the greatest extent) proinflammatory (LTB4), we should consider this method of treatment pathogenetically justified.

943 (FA-247)	Fundamental aspects	GRP under HIPC
Non-contagious BSORP - psoriasis (reflexology)?		

To an even greater extent, the conclusions of researchers of the past years are confirmed by modern new data on the existence of functional systems, as well as by the discovery of new functions of already known systems of the organism.

Hypothetically, it is possible to consider such a mechanism of development of Kebner's phenomenon (and maybe psoriasis in general). There is data (obtained in reflexotherapy practice and researched by scientific method) that the diameter of ATP (active points of reflexotherapy) changes depending on the state of a person: during sleep and in case of strong fatigue their diameter is less than 1 mm; when a person wakes up it increases up to 1 cm;

in the state of emotional tension and in acute diseases, the area of individual ATRs increases even more (even whole areas with increased conductivity are formed).

In essence, ATRs are small areas that contain a complex of interconnected microstructures (vessels, nerves, connective tissue cells) that create a biologically active zone that affects nerve terminals and the communication between these peripheral sites and internal organs. By influencing the ATP, we activate deep sensory pathways. This results in so-called "predictable" sensations that can depend on the stimulation of 5 types of receptors:

1) in the muscle area (receptors are muscle cells);
2) in the area of muscle-tendon transition (receptors - nerve formations of tendons);
3) near the tendon (receptors are lamellar cells);
4) near the articular pouch (type of receptors not identified);
5) in the scalp and other places (receptors - free nerve endings).

It should be remembered that the main scientific concepts of reflexotherapy also to some extent considered the possibility of developing a reflex reaction, depending on the biologically active compounds released during irritation:

1) Tissue therapy theory (action of protein breakdown products and necrohormones that are formed during trauma);
2) the theory of normalising capillary blood flow;
3) Histamine equalisation theory;
4) The chemo-humoral-neural concept (the leading importance is given to prostaglandins, which normalise microcirculation and the functioning of the so-called neuromuscular-vascular unit).

Modern scientists-reflexotherapists note that the mechanisms of influence of reflexotherapy in its basis are similar to the general reflex.

The primary trigger mechanism of reflexotherapy is irritation of receptor formations and subordinate tissues. Stimulation of the receptor apparatus is the beginning of the formation of a feedback reaction of the analyser system, which depends on the degree, nature and duration of stimulation, as well as on the specifically stimulated receptors.

Further impulses on afferent fibres are directed and directed to the leading and associative pathways of the spinal cord.
Depending on which peripheral nerve structures were irritated, the MODALITY OF EXPERIENCED FEELINGS is formed:

1) the sensation of acute local pain is associated with irritation of the A-delta fibres;
2) A diffuse, dull pain sensation depends on C fibres (which slowly conduct nerve impulses);
3) A sensation of heaviness is caused by irritation of receptors that are sensitive to pressure;
4) sensations of pressure - as a result of changes in microcirculation and permeability of the vascular wall, heat - due to increased microcirculation.

That is, at the peripheral level it is a matter of irritation of dermal points and corresponding receptor formations in one way or another. In this case, a local reaction of the ACCON-REFLEX type may develop, with pallor or reddening of the skin near the site of irritation, changes in local temperature, etc. In this case, the microenvironment of receptors (including smooth muscles, blood capillaries, efferent sympathetic fibres) is also changed due to prostaglandins, some enzymes, etc., which are secreted by cells.
The microenvironment of receptors strongly influences their excitation and even makes them more sensitive to other stimuli (the so-called "sensitisation" effect).
At a threshold stimulus value, the segmental apparatus of the spinal cord with the inclusion of fibres of the autonomic nervous system (segmental reaction) is involved in the reverse reaction.
Closely connected vegetative and somatic formations at the level of the spinal cord create prerequisites for switching impulses from the vegetative to the somatic section and vice versa. Direct intersegmental connections between the left and right segments of a segment (associative connections) are also important. Despite the fact that segmental mechanisms are important, the response to stimulation does not end with the segmental reaction alone - a general reaction develops, which includes the main neurohumoral mechanisms of adaptation and homeostasis.

CHAPTER 2

The inflammatory-reparative process - the role of bioelements

It is also known that irritation of postganglionic fibres of the sympathetic nerve renews contractions of transverse striated muscles fatigued by motor nerve irritation. This effect is due to the direct action of the sympathetic nervous system on metabolism and is independent of vascular influence. It is envisaged that this function (adaptation-trophic) in synaptic endings of sympathetic nerves is performed not by neurotransmitters, but by nucleotides, some amino acids, prostaglandins, catecholamines, serotonin and some other biologically active compounds.

944 (FA-248)	Fundamental aspects	GRP under HIPC
Role of bioelements (general information - terminology, classifications)?		

One of the promising directions of scientific research in the coming years will be the study of the role of a particular chemical element both for physiological existence of a particular molecular system and for its "work" under pathological conditions, including the inflammatory-reparative process.

The problem of importance of chemical elements ("chemical language") for vital activity of living organisms has been considered in different years both from the position of science and practical importance in many branches of human activity.

In scientific and practical plan in the greatest degree to the problem of clinical manifestations of toxic influence of those or other microelements on a human organism, attention is paid on chairs of occupational pathology, hygiene and ecology and corresponding clinical bases of higher educational medical institutions (HEMI) and research institutes. Attention is drawn to the fact that the level of microelements that enter the human body can be affected by atmospheric, soil and water pollution, man-made disasters and other factors, the degree of their influence can be very different, even in changes in reproductive function, genetic control and others.

These issues are thoroughly addressed in dentistry as well.

In recent years, a separate scientific and practical direction - bioelemental medicine - has been formed. In this direction, the methods and concepts of such fundamental sciences as physics, chemistry and biology form the basis, and the subject of study is trace elements.

Taking into account the fact that there were many points of view regarding the classification of micronutrients (they were considered as micro-, ultramicro-, macronutrients, etc.), it is considered more appropriate to use a single term - bioelements. In this connection, the term "bioelementosis" was proposed, which is used in cases of deficiency or excess of a microelement in the organism with the development of functional and/or organic disorders. The term "bioelementosis" is understood as a general name of a group of diseases (syndromes), in the pathogenesis of which the leading role is played by certain violations of the microelement composition of the organism. The term

"bioelement metabolism" as an essential indicator of the state of metallo-ligand homeostasis.

BASIC CONCEPTS AND CLASSIFICATIONS. Today there is no universally accepted classification of trace elements, and the term "trace elements" itself should be treated differentiated.

Thus, according to one classification(1st), the chemical element of the human body is divided into:

11 - macronutrients

17 - micronutrients and

22 - ultramicroelement

depending on their concentration (respectively - more than 0.01 %, from 0.00001 % to 0.01 % and up to 0.00001 %).

Of the 11 trace elements, 6 are so-called "organogens" (due to their leading role in forming the structure of tissues and organs).

It is known that the share of only 4 ELEMENTS-ORGANOGENS (oxygen, carbon, hydrogen, nitrogen) accounts for 96 % of human body weight (oxygen - 65 %, nitrogen - 3 %, hydrogen - 10 %, carbon - 18 %), whereas for MACROELEMENTS - 4 %: calcium - 1.7 %, sodium - 0.2 %, chlorine - 0.2 %, sulphur - 0.3 %, phosphorus - 1.25 %, magnesium - 0.05 %, potassium - 0.25 %.

and on MICROELEMENTS - only 0.05 %: fluorine - 0.02 %, iron - 0.006 %, zinc - 0.0033 %; copper, iodine, manganese, cobalt, molybdenum, selenium - 0.0005 %).

The 2nd classification of elements divides them into "structural", "essential" (vital), conditionally essential, toxic, potentially toxic.

The 3rd classification divides elements into 3 groups: those localised in bone tissue, in the reticuloendothelial system and elements that have no tissue specificity.

The 4th classification divides the elements into: vital, probably necessary and elements with a poorly understood role.

In the 5th (modern) classification, the chemical elements are labelled by the new term "ATOMOVITES", and they are divided as follows:

1) in terms of quantitative content in the human body:

1.1) stable;

1.2) permanent;

1.3) temporary;

2) on atomic physiological properties:

2.1) Structural;

2.2) biocatalytic;

2.3) endocrine;

2.4) haematoatomites;

3) on "vital" values for the human body:

3.1) irreplaceable;

3.2) interchangeable;

3.3) understudied;

4) by the intensity of absorption in the GI tract.

As in any other speciality, the large number of classifications shows that they are imperfect.

First things first:

in the organism e really structural trace elements are simultaneously essential, essential - can become toxic, toxic - in low concentrations can be useful;

secondly:

"new-fangled" terms are not always viable, and the "old" term "bioelement" is still the most correct, as it fulfils 3 basic requirements:

1) low toxicity,

2) high digestibility,

3) the form of being in the organism is similar to natural (glycinates, phosphates, citrates, etc.);

third:

an element being in the body in some compound is not always a bioelement, for example:

1) selenium in the form of sodium selenite is not a bioelement, but

selenocysteine or selenomethionine are bioelements;
2) Zinc in the form of sulphate is not a bioelement, but zinc glycinate is a bioelement;
four:
It is envisaged that a free ion (cation, anion) is a transitional form between a chemical element and a bioelement, for example:
1) bioelement - a metal within the metal-ligand complex (metal-amino acid: zinc-aspartate-glycinate);
2) metal-organic acid (potassium citrate, calcium lactate);
3) bioelements are hydrogen and oxygen, which are part of water molecules, nitrogen - which is part of ammonia, etc.
It is still most convenient to use the term bioelements and divide them into:
ORGANOGENS,
MACRO-,
MICRO- and
ULTRAMICROELEMENTS, at that:
- with macronutrients are more related to the ideas of structural functions;
- with trace elements - biochemical and physiological activity is incomparable with their small content in the human body;
- with ultramicroelements - toxicity and insufficient study of their role in the organism.

945 (FA-249)	Fundamental aspects	GRP under HIPC
Role of bioelements (synergism)?		

SYNERGISM. Synergistic elements are those elements that:
1) mutually promote adsorption in the GI tract;
2) help each other in some function at the tissue and cellular levels.
Synergies can be direct or indirect.
Direct synergism:
through phosphorylation processes in the intestinal wall or by influencing the activity of digestive enzymes.
Indirect synergism:

by stimulating the multiplication and activity of microflora in the GI tract.
Synergism can occur at the level of tissue and cellular metabolism:

1) structural interaction

1.1) Ca+P is in bone formation;

1.2) Fe+Cu - in the synthesis of haemoglobin;

1.3) Mg+Zn - in the conformation of RNA molecules in the liver;

2) synergism in the formation of the active centre of the enzyme (iron+copper - as part of cytochrome oxidase);

3) synergy in the activation of enzyme systems and strengthening of the processes of synthesis of substances, activity of endocrine organ function;

4) synergism by mediating effects through hormones on metabolic processes.

946a (FA-250a)	Fundamental aspects	GRP under HIPC
Role of bioelements (antagonism)?		

ANTAGONISM. Antagonists are elements that:

1) inhibit adsorption of each other in the GI tract (magnesium and phosphorus, zinc and copper; the effect of inhibition of adsorption of some elements by others in the GI tract is due to competition for substance-transport ions in the intestinal wall - e.g. Co^{2+}, $Fe2+$);

2) exert an opposite effect on some biochemical function in the body.

Antagonism can be reciprocal or unilateral (calcium inhibits absorption of zinc and magnesium, but there is no feedback).

Such mechanisms of antagonism have been identified:

1) competition of ions for active centres in enzyme systems (divalent magnesium and manganese in metal-enzyme complexes of alkaline phosphatase);

2) competition for binding to a transferrin substance in the blood (divalent iron and zinc are competitors for binding to plasma transferrin).

946b (FA-2506)	Fundamental aspects	GRP under HIPC
The role of bioelements (dynamics in the body)?		

Micronutrients enter the body with food, air and water and in the body they are: assimilated; distributed in tissues; actively functioning (as building materials, as regulators of biochemical processes); excreted from the body.

947 (FA-251)	Fundamental aspects	GRP under HIPC
Role of bioelements (significance of concentration)?		

Dose (concentration) affects the physiological or toxic actions of an element.
Examples:
1) sodium, potassium, calcium, iron, magnesium - in high concentrations can be toxic;
2) Toxic elements such as arsenic, mercury, etc. at low concentrations can be used as drugs.
Therefore, there is a concept of "optimal concentration range", i.e., are necessary for vital functions and, in cases of deficiency or excess, cause serious changes.

948 (FA-252)	Fundamental aspects	GRP under HIPC
Role of bioelements (metal ligand homeostasis)?		

Elements in the body are predominantly in the form of COORDINATION compounds, and their excessive formation or decay leads to disruption of metal ligand homeostasis, and further - to pathology.

949 (FA-253)	Fundamental aspects	GRP under HIPC
Role of bioelements (metal ligand complexes)?		

More than 50% of drugs are potential complexing agents (ligands or metals and their compounds).
Metal-drug complexes can be formed as a result of taking drugs "potential ligands" (so-called endogenous complexes: due to the formation of metals that are part of metalloenzymes).
Coordination compounds of elements are biologically stable, therapeutically effective and safe.
Given that elements, metals and ligands (e.g. ascorbic and linoic acids) can act as both activators and inhibitors of enzymes, it has been possible to create drugs that combine chemical elements with organic substances (ligands).
In addition to their therapeutic value, metal ligand complexes are important components of various diets.

950 (FA-254)	Fundamental aspects	GRP under HIPC
The role of bioelements (the importance of bioelement research)?		

Determination of the content of bioelements in different substrates of the organism has an important informative value regarding the elucidation of various aspects of the pathogenesis of many diseases.
There is a need to compare laboratory and clinical findings and combine them into defined syndromes.
This may be of significant practical importance for diagnosing not only SORP diseases, but also for assessing the clinical condition of patients with injuries to other human systems and organs.

951 (FA-255)	Fundamental aspects	GRP under HIPC
Role of bioelements (responses to damage)?		

Despite the numerous varieties of SORP cellular elements, there are both specific and universal mechanisms of their response to injury.

952 (FA-256)	Fundamental aspects	GRP under HIPC
Role of bioelements (universal reactions)?		

The basis for one of the universal reaction mechanisms of SORP cells is the fundamentally identical structure of their membranes. As a result of damage, the so-called "arachidonic cascade" is triggered, when under the action of cyclooxygenases, lipoxygenases, and epoxygenases, arachidonic acid (biochemical name - eicosatetraenoic acid from "eicose" - 20) is broken down to form so-called eicosanoids (prostaglandins, leukotrienes). The fundamentally identical mechanism of reaction of "defence cells" to damage is also universal: first, endothelial cells of postcapillary venules (treated with cytokines) contract, which allows cellular elements necessary for its elimination and repair of damage to reach the focus of damage. Universal internal information transfer systems also "work" in cells: cAMP/ cGMP, Ca^{2+} , etc. act as second (not secondary !) mediators.

953 (FA-257)	Fundamental aspects	GRP under HIPC
Role of bioelements (principles of BSOPP chronisation)?		

One of the reasons for the chronisation of the course of many BSORPs may be the "programme error" of the normal "sequence" and normal "dose" of inclusion in biochemical processes even one (but most likely several) molecular components of "autocoid" systems. Micronutrients can play an important role in both physiology and pathology of SORP (they are part of molecular systems of perception and processing of information, take part in cascade reactions of inflammatory mediators), their special role is their participation in the processes of antioxidant defence.

954 (FA-258)	Fundamental aspects	GRP under HIPC
The role of bioelements (oxidants)?		

In recent years, the pathogenesis of SARS has been attributed to the importance of OXIDANTS (free radicals), which are molecules or their parts that have an unpaired electron in the molecular (atomic) orbital (i.e., free valence).

They are most often formed during multistep oxidative reactions (as intermediate products), as well as during reactions involving changes in the valence of elements (NADPH, Fe in haemoglobin).

Oxidants (free radicals) include NO_2 (hydropyroxide), RO_2 (peroxide radicals), ***O2*** (superoxide radical), OH (hydroxyl radical), $\backslash O_2$ (singlet oxygen). Hydrogen peroxide, although not a free radical, is actively involved in the formation of OH.

955 (FA-259)	Fundamental aspects	GRP under HIPC
Role of bioelements (free-radical oxidation)?		

FREE RADICAL OXIDATION is a universal physiological process, but excessive accumulation or over-activity of free radicals leads to pathological effects. There are at least 9 known PHYSIOLOGICAL EFFECTS of free radicals:

1) participation in the oxidation and reduction of coenzymes;
2) participation in the transport of oxygen;
3) participation in the processes of tissue respiration;
4) participation in the processes of energy metabolism;
5) Participation in the biosynthesis of progesterone, prostaglandin E_1 , corticosteroids;
6) participation in the construction and self-repair of lipid membrane structures;
7) Acceleration of transmembrane glucose transport;
8) detoxification of xenobiotics (foreign substances);
9) destruction (phagocytosis) of bacteria and viruses.

It is estimated that:

a) 1-3% of inhaled oxygen is used to form superoxidanion and, in this case, each cell in the body produces 10 billion superoxidanion particles daily $(O\ );_2^*$

б) Over the course of a year, the human body produces MORE than 2 KG of superoxide (O_2);

в) Each cell's DNA succumbs to 100,000. Oxidant Shocks per day and MORE than 20 damage.

Repair systems normally repair only 99% of the damage, while 1% of the damage is preserved, and such DNA enters into free-radical branched chain reactions.

956 (FA-260)	Fundamental aspects	GRP under HIPC
Role of bioelements (causes of oxidant formation)?		

There are at least 6 INTERNAL and 9 EXTERNAL causes of excessive free radicals (oxidants).

Among the internal causes (due to the transition of biological oxidation to a non-enzymatic pathway), we can mention such as:

hypovitaminosis
hypoxia
endogenous intoxication
bacterial and viral action
psychoemotional stresses
frequent physical exertion

Among the external causes (oxidant intake from the environment), there are such as:

disturbance of the atmospheric ozone layer;
the effects of penetrating ionising radiation;
radionuclides;
industrial waste;
toxins of non-industrial origin;
substandard products;
tobacco smoke;
alcohol abuse;
Long-term treatment (with chemopreventive drugs, antibiotics, corticosteroids, NSAIDs, painkillers, contraceptives and other medications).

957 (FA-261)	Fundamental aspects	GRP under HIPC
Role of bioelements (pathological effects of free radicals)?		

There are at least 7 known PATHOLOGICAL EFFECTS of excessive accumulation (over-activity) of free radicals:

1) damage to vital enzyme structures of cells with loss of their biological activity:

1.1) succinate dehydrogenase;

1.2) xanthine oxidase (damaged xanthine oxygenase itself becomes an active source of superoxidanion);

1.3) glutathione;

1.4) cytochrome oxidase;

1.5) lipoic acid;

1.6) coenzyme A;

2) initiation of peroxidation of polyunsaturated fatty acids;

3) damage to the lipid component of biological membranes;

4) direct effect on intracellular structures (suppression of cellular immunity, mutations, tumours);

5) suppression of humoral immunity;

6) damage to connective tissue structures;

7) Self-accelerating initiation of the formation of stronger free radicals.

958 (FA-262)	Fundamental aspects	GRP under HIPC
The role of bioelements (antioxidants)?		

In the human body there are SPECIAL substances - ANTIOXIDANTS (antioxidants), which are able to inhibit or eliminate free-radical oxidation of organic substances.

Most of them have a mobile hydrogen atom (AO-C- H). This makes it possible to replace the oxygen in the active free radical and form a low-active radical (radical form of antioxidant).

959 (FA-263)	Fundamental aspects	GRP under HIPC
Role of bioelements (components of AOH)?		

MAIN COMPONENTS OF THE SYSTEM ANTIOXIDANT PROTECTION (AOP) of the body are:

1) biological antioxidants (VITAMINS and other substances that have antioxidant properties);

2) antioxidant FERMENT systems, the activity of which in the majority depends on the place in the active group of the FERMENT:

- Zn,
- C,
- Se
- and other micronutrients.

Thus, micronutrients play an important role in the antioxidant defence system of the body.

960 (FA-264)	Fundamental aspects	GRP under HIPC
Role of bioelements ("trace element" antioxidant enzymes)?		

Thus, at least 7 "MICROELEMENTOSAVISIMABLE" ANTIOXIDANT FERMENTS are known (2 from iron, 2 from copper, and 1 each from zinc, magnesium, and selenium):

1) **Cu-dependent** intracellular superoxide dismutase;
2) **Zn-dependent** intracellular superoxide dismutase;
3) **Mn-dependent** mitochondrial superoxide dismutase;
4) **Fe-dependent** catalase;
5) **Fe-dependent** peroxidase;
6) **Cu-dependent** ceruloplasmin;
7) **Se-dependent** glutathione peroxidase.

Of the above micronutrients that contribute to the synthesis of antioxidant enzymes, selenium and zinc have received the most attention in recent years.

961 (FA-265)	Fundamental aspects	GRP under HIPC
The role of bioelements (mandatory bioelement research)?		

Determination of micronutrient levels in chronic diseases

BSORP is mandatory.

This primarily concerns those of them, in the pathogenesis of which there is an influence of various external factors and concomitant pathology:

1) diseases of the digestive and circulatory organs, etc;
2) nutritional disorders (predominance of carbohydrates and protein deficiency in the diet, the presence of nitrites, nitrates, excessive energy-calorie diet, consumption of foods saturated with extractive substances (rich in cholesterol);
3) focal infection ;
4) hypoxia ;
5) long-term medication;
6) chronic stress (psycho-emotional overstrain, work in extreme or unfavourable climatic conditions);
7) ionising radiation, excessive infrared or ultraviolet irradiation, unfavourable industrial and environmental situation;
8) tobacco smoking, alcohol abuse.

962 (FA-266)	Fundamental aspects	GRP under HIPC
Role of bioelements (mandatory bioelement studies - under which BSOPPs)?		

Disorders of the body's bioelemental composition, which affects antioxidant enzymes, are seen in virtually everyone patients with diseases that affect the SORP: psoriasis, pyoderma, candidiasis, allergies, red squamous lichen planus, fungal and viral diseases; pre-tumour and tumour diseases of the SORP, etc.

The above dictates the need for new research on bioelements in dental practice.

The data obtained can confidently testify to the syndromic nature of lesions in SARS.

963 (FA-267)	Fundamental aspects	GRP under HIPC
The role of bioelements (SORP and bioelements - general information)?		

SORP is not only a powerful receptor field, performs a number of immune and endocrine functions, but also participates in the metabolism of bioelements.

Protein-energy insufficiency , deficit
micronutrients (zinc, copper, iron), vitamins (retinol, ascorbic acid, alpha-tocopherol, folic acid), as well as ionising radiation and impaired neurohumoral regulation are among the important causes of secondary immunodeficiency.

964 (FA-268)	Fundamental aspects	GRP under HIPC
Role of bioelements (non-specificity of bioelement changes)?		

Studies by means of atomic emission and adsorption spectrometry of trace elements content in a number of BSOPPs showed that symptoms of different BSOPPs have non-specific significance (identical changes in different BSOPPs are detected).

So, in the presence of:

1) pyoderma is noted :

J Deficit:

- chroma
- selena
- zinc
- manganese
- silicon
- potassium
- sodium

- sulphur ***J*** excess:
- copper
- iodine;

2) inflammation, irritation and dryness of SORP, respectively : ***J*** deficiency:

- zinc
- selena
- silicon
- sulphur
- calcium
- potassium

J surplus:

- arsenic
- chroma
- nickel
- cobalt
- copper
- cadmium;

3) pigmentation disorders of certain areas of the SORP, respectively:

J Deficit:

- copper
- manganese
- selena
- silicon
- potassium
- sodium
- zinc ***J*** excess:
- arsenic
- copper
- lead
- cadmium;

4) allergic manifestations, respectively:

J Deficit:

- selena
- zinc
- calcium
- silicon
- manganese

J surplus:

- - chroma
- nickel
- cobalt
- arsenic
- cadmium
- lead
- iodine.

Taking into account that correction of such disorders without previous bioelemental examination is ineffective, and at present there are still difficulties in bioelemental diagnostics, it is recommended that patients should be fed with consideration of the bioelemental evaluation of certain products.

965 (FA-269)	Fundamental aspects	GRP under HIPC
Role of bioelements (The role of bioelemental assessment of foods)?		

1. It was found that the most effective blocker of caesium absorption[137] is ferrocin (potassium iron hexacyanoferrate). It is also known that a sufficient amount of iron and potassium is found in apples, legumes, brewer's yeast, and corn. In this regard, it is recommended that patients should include these foods in their diet, especially since their use is also pathogenetically justified in the abovementioned SORP lesions.
2. Due to the fact that calcium is an analogue of strontium, then to reduce the pathological effects of strontium and caesium usually use appropriate blockers and/or decorporants. At the same time, with such treatment there is a risk of disturbance of metabolism of the strontium analogue calcium. In order to avoid calcium imbalance in the organism, patients are recommended to eat foods that contain calcium in the highest quantity (leafy vegetables, parsley, spinach, millet, oat and pearl cereals, milk, cheese).
3. The radioprotective and general therapeutic effects of seaweed products are known - their inclusion in the diet reduces the accumulation of caesium[137] and strontium[85] , and in children who live in contaminated areas, they contribute to a more intensive excretion of radionuclides.

Therefore, these products are also recommended to appropriate patients, as they simultaneously contain calcium, iron, copper, magnesium, manganese, selenium, silicon and iodine. The importance of these elements in SORP changes has been outlined above, and in the presence of thyroid function disorders in the majority of patients in this category, all the more justifies the inclusion of appropriate foods in the diet.

4. Alimentary prophylaxis of the long-term effects of radiation should be based on the reduction of lipid peroxidation. These processes are the basis of pathophysiological mechanisms of radiation action and need appropriate nutritional correction. It has been established that selenium is a natural antioxidant, and iron, zinc and cobalt are important stimulators of hematopoiesis.
5. Selenium is found in some of the above foods (spinach, legumes, cheese, seaweed) as well as in meat, walnuts and olive oil, which necessitates appropriate dietary recommendations.
6. Zinc and cobalt are contained in buckwheat, millet groats, rice and it is also recommended that patients include the corresponding products in their diet.

966 (FA-270)	Fundamental aspects	GRP under HIPC
The role of bioelements (bioelemental syndromes)?		

The study of bioelement composition of patients with chronic BSOPP made it possible to reveal a number of nonspecific changes, which, however, indicate a certain "bioelement syndrome" of some of them.

Determination of the content of trace elements in individuals who live in areas of environmental risk indicates the possibility of using the method of atomic emission and adsorption spectrometry to determine disorders of the so-called "metal-ligand" homeostasis.

Data on these abnormalities can to some extent be used as markers for further examination of patients to identify neoplastic, precancerous or paraneoplastic processes in them.

967 (FA-271)	Fundamental aspects	GRP under HIPC

Role of bioelements (bioelementosis in precancrosis and cancer)?

Atypical course (so-called "precancroses", "paraneoplastic processes") is also among the potentially dangerous in terms of cancer. The data have been obtained, which allow us to suggest that the propensity to neoplastic processes is observed in :

deficits:

- zinc
- iron
- cobalt
- manganese
- selena

and excess:

- arsenic
- nickel
- chroma
- beryllium
- copper
- lead
- cadmium
- vanadium
- of mercury,
- cobalt.

With respect to calcium, evidence shows that any abnormalities in its content in the body may contribute to a propensity for cancer.

These data require further careful analysis in the light of such important circumstances:

1) copper, in spite of the fact that its excess is determined in patients with "oncoprofile", is still used (along with selenium and zinc) as a micronutrient immunotherapy as an additional technique to chemotherapy for patients with various forms of cancer;

2) Among the numerous functions of calcium, there is also its important role as a "universal second mediator" for the transmission of most information signals into the cell (even other second mediator systems, such as cAMP, cGMP, etc., depend on its functioning);

3) Zinc in general is an element that needs to be studied extensively,

given that according to various data it is a component of more than 200 enzymes or more than 300 zinc-containing proteins; taking into account its influence on transcription processes, its intervention in regulatory processes involved in tumour disease (similar to cytokines) can be considered.

968 (FA-272)	Fundamental aspects	GRP under HIPC
Role of bioelements (eczematous BSORPs - relevance)?		

Despite many years of research into the pathogenesis of eczema, and even the use of the latest technologies in modern medicine, there are still many open questions that need more detailed and in-depth study. Improvement and development of new and more effective methods of treatment of this disease also remains relevant. There is an increase in the frequency of sensitisation of the organism to a wide variety of food products along with the expansion of the arsenal of so-called "allergenic food" (which is predetermined mainly by violations of cooking technologies and quite frequent use of ingredients of "dubious" quality, inclusion of preservatives, dyes and other chemical compounds, which most often become the causes of both the emergence and exacerbation of existing hypersensitivity of the organism). Among the environmental causes, the advantage is left by the consequences of the Chernobyl accident, harmful ~ 92 ~ industrial emissions into the atmosphere, the level of which in recent years is continuously increasing.

Despite the saturation of the pharmaceutical market with a large number of (including - quite new) drugs, developments of leading companies regarding the treatment of eczematous BSOPP, and taking into account the above-mentioned features of eczema, the problem of etiology, mechanisms of development, its therapy is still quite relevant and needs further research.

According to many scientists, special attention should be paid to non-medicamentous methods of treatment, which include phytotherapy, as well as the use of mineral complexes. At the same time, chronotherapy methods are rarely used, i.e. taking into account physiological circadian and seasonal biorhythms of the human body.

It is urgent to improve the methods of treatment of patients with true eczema on the basis of studying the role of essential elements and indicators of lipid peroxidation (LPO) and antioxidant defence (AOD), determining their role in the pathogenesis of the disease.

969 (FA-273)	Fundamental aspects	GRP under HIPC
Role of bioelements (eczematous BSORPs - role of essential bioelements)?		

In patients with true eczema the uranium of essential elements (Fe - iron, I - iodine, Si - copper, Mn - manganese, Zn - zinc, Co - cobalt, Mo - molybdenum, Se - selenium, Cr - chromium, V - vanadium) were studied; their deficiency was revealed in all patients.

970 (FA-274)	Fundamental aspects	GRP under HIPC
The role of bioelements (bioelements and enzymeopathies)?		

Biomarkers (Co, Fe, Cu, Zn) of metal ligand homeostasis disturbance (activation of POL processes and imbalance of AOS) were determined on the basis of bioelement changes in patients with true eczema.
As mentioned above, among all trace elements, a special group includes the so-called essential (indispensable), the regular intake of which is absolutely necessary for the body's normal vital activity.
These include: Fe, J, Si, Mn, Mn, Zn, Co, Mo, Se, Cg, V.
Among the many causes that can cause micronutrient deficiency (nutritional, GI diseases, bad habits, etc.), an important place belongs to chronic psycho-emotional stress.
The presence of rashes on the SOPR and skin, almost constant itching, poor efficacy of treatment are stress factors for eczema patients.
Regardless of the etiological factor that causes chronic deficiency of essential trace elements in the pathogenesis of various pathological conditions arising in this case, the key role belongs to enzymeopathies.
Micronutrients can be directly incorporated into the structure of the enzyme molecule (catalytic centre), or act as coenzymes, be electron

acceptors or donors.

Each micronutrient plays its own unique role in metabolic processes.

Since micronutrients are not synthesised in the body, the normal course of biochemical processes is directly dependent on external input, and if it is insufficient, they should be supplemented .

971 (FA-275)	Fundamental aspects	GRP under HIPC
Role of bioelements (efficacy of integrated therapy)?		

Pathogenetically substantiated complex therapy of patients with true eczema with simultaneous use of polymicroelemental agent (e.g., Esmin®) and phytoantioxidant (e.g., Baikal hellebore extract, taking into account the circadian biorhythm of "adrenal cortex hormone secretion").

The effectiveness of this method of treatment was proved (absence of relapses or less severity of their manifestations; normalisation of indices of bioelements, POL and AOS enzymes changed before treatment).

It should be noted that in this method 3 types of biorhythms were taken into account: circadian ("secretion of adrenal cortex hormones"); seasonal (prophylactic courses in spring and autumn) and, so to say, "pharmacokinetic" (constituents of modern drugs like esmin are absorbed in a certain chronological order each when entering the body).

The results of the clinical effect had a direct correlative dependence on the dynamics of the indicators of the study of metalloligand homeostasis, POL and AOH enzymes.

972 (FA-276)	Fundamental aspects	GRP under HIPC
Role of bioelements (action of polymicroelemental preparation - Esmin)?		

ESMIN is an original polymicroelement preparation, which is manufactured in Ukraine. Composition of the drug:

- iron - 3 mg
- zinc - 4 mg

- manganese - 0.8 mg
- copper - 0.7 mg
- cobalt - 0.07 mg
- chromium - 0.07 mg
- selenium - 0.05 mg
- molybdenum - 0.07 mg
- vanadium - 0.01 mg
- mefenamic acid - 85 mg

Mephenamic acid is a very important component, because it forms chelate complexes with microelements, which ensures optimal absorption of the drug components in the GI tract. This acid has an independent action - as an inducer of endogenous interferon. Especially important is the fact that Esmin is a purely "microelemental" preparation (not combined with vitamins). Some vitamins and minerals are known to block each other's absorption in the GI tract (competition for common transport systems). Due to the wide range of positive biological effects, the field of clinical application of esmin is extremely wide. It should also be considered appropriate to take esmin for preventive purposes (to increase the body's resistance to the influence of unfavourable environmental factors, to strengthen adaptive capabilities).

973 (FA-277)	Fundamental aspects	GRP under HIPC
Role of bioelements (action of phytoantioxidants)?		

BAIKAL SHLEMNIK (SB) is one of the preparations used for eczema. The medicinal properties of SB were noticed many centuries ago in Tibet and China. Pharmacologists primarily point to folk medicine data on the sedative and hypotensive properties of SWB, as well as to the
its use during wars, due to frequent stresses that led to neuroses and high blood pressure (which is especially relevant today).
The roots and rhizomes of SWB contain
flavonoids:

- baicalin
- baicalein
- wagonin

- skutelarein

saponins

essential oils

alkaloids

starch

tannins

resins

Flavonoids account for the wide range of medicinal properties of sloeberry:

baicalin inhibits lipid peroxidation 375 times more strongly than vitamin E

flavonoid vagonin shows neuroprotective and anxiolytic action, having a pronounced affinity for the active benzodiazepine centres of GABAergic receptors This and other features can explain the multifaceted mechanism of action of flavonoids.

CHAPTER 3

Inflammatory-reparative process - in purulent lesions of SORP and wounds

Antioxidant properties of ShB are so powerful that they allow it to be successfully used even in the treatment of patients with oncopathology who have received chemotherapy and radiotherapy.
ShB contains not only flavonoids, but also steroidal saponins (7 %), which possess adaptogenic properties, regulate water-salt and mineral metabolism, have anti-inflammatory effect, are used in atherosclerosis, enhance the activity of hormones, enzymes, due to emulsifying effect, are used as diuretic, laxative means, as well as - as a source of synthesis of corticosteroids. With careful study in experiment, not only anti-inflammatory, but also anti-allergic action of this drug, as well as its antithrombic and antibacterial properties have been proved.

974 (FA-278)	Fundamental aspects	GRP in SORP Pus lesions and RANACH.
Etiology?		

Normally, the microbiocenosis of superficial tissues involves colonisation by gram-positive bacteria (Propionibacterium, Corynebacterium, epidermal staphylococci, micrococci, streptococci, as well as yeast-like fungi and, less frequently, transient microflora). With decreased immunity, the number of gram-negative bacteria increases. Such microorganisms as staphylococci, streptococci, pneumococci, Escherichia coli, Proteus vulgaris, Pseudomonas bacillus, etc. can be the cause of purulent lesions of SORP.
The leading role in the occurrence of such acute processes belongs to staphylococci and streptococci, in the development of deep and chronic - mixed infection with the addition of gram-negative flora.

975 (FA-279)	Fundamental aspects	GRP in SORP Pus lesions and RANACH.

Classification of suppurative lesions of SORP?

All purulent lesions of SORP are divided into primary (occur on the unchanged surface) and secondary (develop against the background of damage to SORP or as manifestations of a complicated course of other pathology.

Streptococcal lesions usually occur in the presence of microtrauma, and staphylococcal lesions in intact areas. The likelihood of colonisation increases in the presence of allergic diseases.

These processes are also divided into uncomplicated and complicated (the course of which becomes more severe with the involvement of other tissues in the pathological process and dictates the need for surgical intervention).

Despite certain disadvantages of the above classification, it is not only convenient in practical terms, but also really corresponds to reality.

976 (FA-280)	Fundamental aspects	GRP in SORP Pus lesions and RANACH.
Modern differences?		

In recent years, there has been an increase in the number of cases of chronic course of purulent lesions of SORP, in which a low degree of isolation of etiological pathogens from the lesions is noted.

This is primarily due to inadequate and uncontrolled use of antibiotics, which do not kill bacteria, but promote their transformation into L-forms.

Such forms lose their typical properties, but retain the main feature - the ability to cause disease.

The result of bacterial transformation into L-forms is the formation of bacillus carriers and bacterial variants with high drug resistance, as well as chronic and atypical forms of diseases.

977 (FA-281)	Fundamental aspects	GRP in SORP Pus lesions and RANACH.
Features of the morphology of the pathogens?		

A distinctive feature of the main causative agents of purulent inflammatory processes in humans (gram-positive cocci: staphylo- and streptococci) is the absence of the ability to spore formation, spherical shape, positive Gram staining.

978 (FA-282)	Fundamental aspects	GRP in SORP and Wound Pus Injuries
Staphylococcus aureus - specifics?		

Staphylococcus aureus is everywhere but the skin.
colonise the surfaces of mucous membranes.
Since their detection from human purulent lesions, their property of forming clusters that resemble bunches of grapes has been noted, which became the basis of their name. They form rounded colonies of cream, yellow or orange colour when cultured under aerobic conditions. It is these lipochromic pigments that protect staphylococci from the action of toxic oxygen radicals.

979 (FA-283)	Fundamental aspects	GRP in SORP Pus Infections and RANACH.
Staphylococci - what do they cause?		

Some staphylococci are representatives of the normal microflora of the skin and mucous membranes of humans, others are cause purulent processes, abscesses, various biogenic infections and even fatal septicaemia. Enterotoxin produced by some staphylococci causes food poisoning.

980 (FA-284)	Fundamental aspects	GRP in SORP Pus Infections and RANACH.
Are staphylococci antigenic substances?		

Staphylococcus aureus has more than 50 antigenic substances, many of which are allergens. Species-specific antigens are teichoic acids and protein A for Staphylococcus aureus.

981 (FA-285)	Fundamental aspects	GRP in SORP and Wound Pus Injuries
Staphylococcus aureus groups?		

Depending on the presence of coagulase, staphylococci are divided into 2 groups, among which human diseases are caused by both coagulase-positive and coagulase-negative species, i.e. pathogenic staphylococci cause haemolysis of erythrocytes and coagulation of plasma.

982 (FA-286)	Fundamental aspects	GRP in SORP Pus lesions and RANACH.
Streptococci - specifics?		

Ever since the isolation of streptococci in rye, wound infections, and septicaemia, it has been noted that these pathogens parasitise surfaces (including SORPs), and in smears they are arranged in pairs, or short chains, from which they derive their name.

In 1884, Rosenbach introduced the name S. p yogenes.

983 (FA-287)	Fundamental aspects	GRP in SORP and Wound Pus Injuries
Streptococci - activity?		

The characteristic features of streptococci are not only the absence of catalase activity, but also the ability to lysis erythrocytes. Depending on their haemolytic activity, they are divided into alpha-haemolytic (partial haemolysis), beta-haemolytic (complete haemolysis) and gamma-haemolytic (no haemolysis) species; beta-haemolytic streptococci are the main causative agents of human diseases.

984 (FA-288)	Fundamental aspects	GRP in SORP and Wound Pus Injuries
The causative agents of suppurative lesions - pathogenic properties?		

The pathogenic properties of a particular strain of purulent pathogens are determined by the sum of extracellular factors, toxins, and the invasiveness of a particular strain and vary considerably. Adhesins are surface proteins that interact with proteoglycans of connective tissue and proteins of extracellular marix.

985 (FA-289)	Fundamental aspects	GRP in SORP Pus lesions and RANACH.
The causative agents of purulent lesions - pathogenicity factors (microcapsule)?		

The pathogenicity factors of the above pathogens are microcapsule, cell wall components, enzymes and toxic substances.

Regarding the microcapsule, it should be noted that it:

protects the pathogen from complement-mediated uptake by neutrophils

promotes adhesion of the pathogen

helps it spread through the tissues

986 (FA-290)	Fundamental aspects	GRP in SORP and Wound Pus Injuries
The causative agents of purulent lesions - pathogenicity factors (cell wall components)?		

Cell wall components as pathogenicity factors:

stimulate the development of inflammatory reactions (increase the synthesis of interleukin-1 by macrophages)

activate the complement system

are potent chemoattractants for neutrophils.

987 (FA-291)	Fundamental aspects	GRP in SORP Pus Infections and RANACH.
Are pathogenicity factors (teichoic acids) the causative agents of purulent lesions?		

Teichoic acids as pathogenicity factors:
start an alternative pathway of the complementary cascade
activate the coagulation and kallikrein-kinin systems
facilitate adhesion to epithelial surfaces
may inhibit the absorptive activity of phagocytes

988 (FA-292)	Fundamental aspects	GRP in SORP and Wound Pus Injuries
The causative agents of purulent lesions - pathogenicity factors (protein A)?		

Protein A as a pathogenicity factor:
nonspecifically binds the Fc fragment of IgG (which activates complement components through both alternative and classical pathways)
enhances the activity of natural killer cells
exhibits superatigenic properties, which together with complement activation leads to various local and systemic reactions (suppression of phagocyte activity, etc.).

989 (FA-293)	Fundamental aspects	GRP in SORP Pus lesions and RANACH.
Are pathogenicity factors (complement activation) the causative agents of purulent lesions?		

Complement activation leads to a variety of local and systemic reactions:
anaphylaxis

Arthus phenomenon
inhibition of phagocyte activity, etc.

990 (FA-294)	Fundamental aspects	GRP in SORP and Wound Pus Injuries
Are pathogenicity factors (enzymes) the causative agents of purulent lesions?		

Enzymes exert a variety of influences:

- catalase protects bacteria from the action of oxygen-dependent microbocidal mechanisms of phagocytosis
- beta-lactamase breaks down beta-lactam antibiotic molecules
- lipases facilitate adhesion and tissue penetration
- Coagulase exists in 3 antigenic forms:

o causes the serum to clot

o does not interact directly with fibrinogen, but forms a thrombin-like substance, which possibly interacts with prothrombin as well

991 (FA-295)	Fundamental aspects	GRP in SORP Pus Infections and RANACH.
Are pathogenicity factors (haemolysins) causative agents of purulent lesions?		

There are 4 antigenic types of haemolysins that are capable of causing complete haemolysis:

- alpha-haemolysin (alpha-toxin) inactive in
against human erythrocytes, but when administered to animals it causes necrotic reactions and their deaths
- beta-haemolysin (sphingomyelinase) performs
moderate effect on human erythrocytes, exhibits pronounced cold haemolysis properties
- gamma-haemolysin (two-component haemolysin) has moderate activity against haemolysis of red blood cells.
- delta haemolysin is an aggregate of low molecular weight compounds

that exhibit detergent properties (i.e., can cause broad-spectrum cytotoxicity).

992 (FA-296)	Fundamental aspects	GRP in SORP Pus lesions and RANACH.
The causative agents of purulent lesions - pathogenicity factors (toxins)?		

Toxins include:

- exfoliatins A and B - cause the development of burnt skin syndrome
- toxic shock syndrome toxin - responsible for the development of a specific symptom complex (primarily due to stimulation of tumour necrosis factor release).
- delta-toxin (leucocidin) - inhibits water absorption and activates the formation of cAMP (which is important in staphylococcal diarrhoea; has a cytotoxic effect on polymorphonuclear leucocytes).
- enterotoxin A-F - responsible for the development of food intoxications

993 (FA-297)	Fundamental aspects	GRP in SORP and Wound Pus Injuries
Are the causative agents of purulent lesions pathogenicity factors ("sensitisers")?		

Many components of staphylococci and their metabolites have a sensitising effect, which is manifested in reactions of immediate or delayed types and the development of relevant clinical changes, including on the SOPP.

994 (FA-298)	Fundamental aspects	GRP in SORP and Wound Pus Injuries
Are streptococci immune response factors?		

Such factors have many features in common with the immune response to bacterial infections of other etiologies, and among such that influence the response are:

- patient's age
- immune status
- history of contact with a streptococcal pathogen (primarily beta-haemolytic group A streptococcus)

It is assumed that the more severe course of streptococcal infection in older age is due to preliminary sensitisation of the immune system to this pathogen (more pronounced immune response to the action of bacterial toxins and enzymes).

995 (FA-299)	Fundamental aspects	GRP in SORP and Wound Pus Injuries
Are streptococci the surface components of the wall?		

Streptococcal antigens are represented not only by specific toxins (streptolysins O and S, exotoxin) and enzymes (hyaluronidase and streptokinase), but also surface components of the bacterial wall (M protein, hyaluronic acid).

It should be emphasised that as a result of the damaging effect of specific toxins on cells (in particular leukocytes), specific enzymes are released that enhance the development and prevalence of inflammatory reactions, but M protein has the greatest immunogenicity.

996 (FA-300)	Fundamental aspects	GRP in SORP Pus lesions and RANACH.
Streptococci - antibodies to antigens?		

Antibodies to streptococcal antigens that appear on the 4-6th day are not important in elimination of the pathogen and slowing down of the pathological process, but determination of the level of antibodies to streptolysin-O (antistreptolysin-O) and to deoxyribonuclease-B (anti-DNA-ase-B) is informative in diagnosing the localisation of the pathological process.

In particular, the level of the former increases with infection in the nasopharynx, and with an increase in both types of antibodies - the pathological process is localised in the skin.

997 (FA-301)	Fundamental aspects	GRP in SORP Pus Infections and RANACH.
Are streptococci antibodies to exotoxin?		

Streptococcal exotoxin, acting as a polyclonal activator of B-lymphocytes, is a powerful stimulator of the immune response, activating a significant number of B-lymphocytes, thus leading to an increase in antibody (immunoglobulin) synthesis and serum levels, which is observed in chronic diseases. In fact, antigen-specific stimulation causes only activation of specific antibodies and cannot significantly affect the level of immunoglobulins in serum.

998 (FA-302)	Fundamental aspects	GRP in SORP Pus Infections and RANACH.
The causative agents of suppurative lesions - a phenomenon of "slippage"?		

One of the factors for bacteria in the body to survive (the so-called "evasion" phenomenon from the immune response) is the presence of certain structures and functions in them.

So, for example:

- polysaccharide capsule - prevents phagocytosis
- mucus secretion - reduces activation of complement system components via alternative pathway
- antigenic variation is an example of relapsing fever in boreliosis infection
- proteases - reduce the activity and destroy secretory immunoglobulin A
- infected cells with weak phagocytic activity - contribute to long-term persistence of the pathogen

999 (FA-303)	Fundamental aspects	GRP in SORP and Wound Pus Injuries

The causative agents of suppurative lesions - mechanisms of injury?

Damage to organs and tissues accompanied by the death of host cells is the result of the action of toxins that produce bacteria, as well as the processes of hyperactivation of the immune system in response to the introduction of pathogens.

At the same time, it can be quite difficult to identify a single mechanism of damage. A striking example of this is streptococcal infection (hypersensitivity to beta- haemolytic streptococcus can lead to the development of rheumatism, post-streptococcal glomerulonephritis, and erythema nodosum).

1000 (FA-304)	Fundamental aspects	GRP in SORP Pus Infections and RANACH.
The causative agents of suppurative lesions - nature of the lesion?		

Endogenous character of damage have the majority of diseases that are caused by staphylococcus, and the mechanism of infection is more often associated with the transfer of the pathogen from the sites of colonisation on the injured surface (but a significant role may also play a close contact with persons who suffer from staphylococcal diseases, as well as with carriers of staphylococci).

For example, in adults, Staphylococcus aureus is isolated in 15-50% of healthy individuals, and temporary carriage in 60%.

Chronic carriage is typical for staff of medical institutions, patients who suffer from atopic diseases, as well as in persons who receive injections of various drugs (diabetics, drug addicts, etc.).

Epidermal staphylococci, which normally colonise certain areas of the skin, can also colonise mucous membranes. They are members of the normal microflora not only of the human skin, but also of the respiratory tract and the alimentary tract and are constantly found in the air and the environment. They are identified in patients with reduced resistance. Most often they are the cause of injuries caused by infection of various devices (prostheses, catheters), or there is haematogenous dissemination of the pathogen after surgical interventions.

1001 (FA-305)	Fundamental aspects	GRP in SORP Pus lesions and RANACH.
Are the causative agents of suppurative lesions extra-hospital and nosocomial infections?		

The causative agents of wound purulent infections are
The majority of bacteremias, pneumonias, and infectious lesions of various tissues are causative agents of a significant proportion of out-of-hospital and nosocomial bacteremias, pneumonias, and infectious lesions of various tissues.
Of particular importance is the spread of staphylococci, which are resistant or have reduced sensitivity to modern antibiotics. They easily develop resistance to many antimicrobials, which creates great difficulties in the treatment of patients.
These features are the reason for a significant limitation in the choice of antibacterial agents for the treatment of infections caused by these strains of microorganisms.

1002 (FA-306)	Fundamental aspects	GRP in SORP Pus lesions and RANACH.
The causative agents of suppurative lesions - problematic aspects of treatment?		

Due to the fact that isolation of purulent infection pathogens and determination of their sensitivity to antibiotics is not always available and cost-effective, the treatment of such patients is usually empirical, which often leads to complications of the course of diseases. The growth of resistance of purulent infections pathogens to antibacterial drugs (which depends, among other things, on their irrational and uncontrolled use) is of particular concern in modern times.

1003 (FA-307)	Fundamental aspects	GRP in SORP and Wound Pus Injuries
The causative agents of suppurative lesions - antibiotic therapy?		

In modern times, there are many recommendations for antibiotic therapy of purulent infections and, for example, in such a disease (including SORP) as impetigo, it is recommended to use:

- cloxacillin, cephalexin, co-trimoxazole
- if the causative agent is pyogenic streptococcus - penicillin, erythromycin, mupirocin, cephalosporins
- if the causative agent is Staphylococcus aureus - cloxacillin, dicloxacillin, mupirocin, cephalosporins

1004 (FA-308)	Fundamental aspects	GRP in SORP and Wound Pus Injuries
The causative agents of suppurative lesions - antibiotic resistance?		

Resistance to the following antibiotics has been established against Staphylococcus aureus:

- to erythromycin - 49.4 per cent
- to chloramphenbicol, 32%.
- to ciprofloxacin - 23.1%
- to lincomycin - 21.1%
- to clindamycin - 16.5 per cent
- to tetracycline - 8.9%
- to gentamicin in 8%

For current antibiotics, evidence of minor (1-5%) resistance of staphylococci to mucopyrocin and fusidic acid has been reported, but there are increasing reports of increasing resistance to methicillin.

Significantly complicates the choice of treatment tactics for patients and the development of multidrug resistance.

1004 (FA-308)	Fundamental aspects	GRP in SORP and Wound Pus Injuries
The causative agents of suppurative lesions - antibiotic resistance?		

The pathogenic properties of a particular strain of pustular pathogen and resistance to cantibiotics may be determined by the combined effect of :

- extracellular factors
- toxins
- the invasive properties of a particular strain
- the different pathogenicity of different strains

1005 (FA-309)	Fundamental aspects	GRP in SORP and Wound Pus Injuries
The causative agents of suppurative lesions - highly accurate methods for resistance diagnosis?		

Resistant to etiotropic therapy strains of pustular pathogens, which have spread in the

Recently, the low availability of high-precision methods for determining such resistance (multiprimer PCR and other methods of genetic identification of antibiotic-resistant strains of staphylococci and streptococci), the great importance of endogenous factors in the development of such infections necessitates the introduction of methods of immunomodulatory therapy for the patients concerned.

1006 (FA-310)	Fundamental aspects	GRP in SORP and Wound Pus Injuries
Are the causative agents of purulent lesions extracellular adhesive proteins?		

Factors of intercellular relationships are important for the virulence of pustular pathogens, and play a significant role in the pathogenesis of the respective diseases caused by these microorganisms.

For example, the extracellular adhesive protein of Staphylococcus aureus is an analogue of the major histocompatibility complex, as it has high affinity to various proteins of the organism (fibronectin, fibrinogen, thrombospondin, etc.); it takes part in the regulation of the inflammatory response through interaction with intracellular adhesion molecules ICAM-1.

1007 (FA-311)	Fundamental aspects	GRP in SORP Pus Infections and RANACH.
Are the causative agents of suppurative lesions other molecular systems?		

Other molecular systems that ensure adhesion of bacteria to certain tissues may also play a role as virulence factors. For example, for Staphylococcus aureus, these are:

- collagen-binding protein - not expressed in most strains, mediates bacterial adhesion to collagen and plays an active role in the pathogenesis of many purulent infections.
- Agglutinating factors A and B bind fibrinogen, with factor A mediating platelet aggregation and fibrin clot formation, which are initiated by Staphylococcus aureus
- Elastin-binding protein is involved in bacterial colonisation by binding to elastin and is present in the tissues of some organs and blood vessel walls.
- Fibronectin-binding proteins promote Staphylococcus aureus adhesion by binding to fibronectin and may function as an invasion factor
- intracellular adhesive proteins are involved in biofilm formation, allowing bacteria to attach to each other, as well as to body tissues
- Proteins that contain serine-asparagine are involved in bacterial adhesion through the binding of bone tissue sialoprotein

1008 (FA-312)	Fundamental aspects	GRP in SORP and Wound Pus Injuries

Are fibronectin-binding proteins the causative agents of purulent lesions?

Streptococci that produce this factor are able to colonise collagen, which provides them with protection against adhesion by polymorphonuclear leukocytes in the presence of opsonising antibodies.

These same adhesive molecules bind fibronectin, which results in the movement of matrix into the space between streptococcal cells and favours the formation of large bacterial aggregates.

1009 (FA-313)	Fundamental aspects	GRP in SORP and Wound Pus Injuries
Are the causative agents of suppurative lesions factors of bacterial adhesion to tissues?		

If they are considered by the example of S. ryogenes, they include:

- antiproteolysis is performed by the G-related alpha-2-macroglobulin-binding protein by
binding of the protease inhibitor alpha-2-macroglobulin to the surface of the bacterial cell, inhibiting proteolysis while protecting M-protein and other cell surface structures.
- antiphagocytosis is carried out due to hyaluronic acid of the capsule (protection from phagocytosis occurs by so-called masking of the bacterial cell) and M-protein (prevents complement activation through alternative pathway and phagocytosis by binding complement activating factors and fibrinogen. M-protein (prevents complement activation through alternative pathway and phagocytosis by binding complement activating factors and fibrinogen; it is a mediator of adhesion to epitheliocytes and it is believed that M-protein takes part in the development of inflammatory response - binding of fibrinogen, kinogen or plasminogen).
- streptococcal inhibitor of complement-mediated lysis, binding to the insertion site of complement, inhibits lysis of bacterial cells; inhibits synthesis of mucosal protective factors - lysozyme, secretory leukocyte protease inhibitor, human alpha-defensin-1 and cathelicidin
- complement protease C5a-peptidase promotes bacterial proliferation and damages the chemotactic factor of this complement, which prevents neutrophils from migrating to the focus of infection.
- The extracellular enzyme DNAase is a factor of invasion, damages

DNA that is released from dead cells, reduces the viscosity of the pus and allows greater mobility of the microorganism

- hyaluronidase is an invasion factor, damages hyaluronic acid as a component of connective tissue, favours the spread of bacteria
- IgG-damaging enzyme inhibits phagocytosis by protecting bacteria from opsonising IgG antibodies
- Streptococcal pyrogenic exotoxin B facilitates bacterial proliferation and survival, induces inflammatory response
- The plasminogen activator is streptokinase, which is also a tissue invasion factor
- streptolysin-O is a toxin that damages cells with cholesterol in their membranes; in subcellular concentrations, it affects phagocyte function by increasing cytokine secretion and inducing cell apoptosis.
- streptolysin-S lyses a wide range of cells, including lymphocytes and neutrophils

- Pyrogenic exotoxins cause the development of streptococcal toxic shock syndrome and scarlatina, and play a role in autoimmune reactions after streptococcal infections.

1010 (FA-314)	Fundamental aspects	GRP in SORP Pus lesions and RANACH.
Immune response - suppressors?		

The discoveries of Th1, Th2, Th3, Threg have raised doubts about the existence of suppressors as a separate unit of immune cells. There is increasing evidence that this function is specific to certain cytokines, which may be of different cellular origin.

However, CD8+ cells retain this capability (i.e., synthesis of suppressor cytokines). In addition, it was found that there is a structure (CD28) on the surface of these cells, which clearly allows to distinguish 2 phenotypes - CD8+CD28+ (T-killer) and CD8+CD28- (T-suppressor).

The CD4+/CD8+ ratio is included in the three main features of the so-called "immunological risk phenotype", i.e., the immunodeficiency state of a particular person:

J accumulation of CD4+CD28- T-lymphocyte suppressors

J decrease in the CD4+/CD8+ T-cell ratio less than unity

J decreased proliferative capacity of T-lymphocytes to mitogens

Thus, the existence of CD8+ T cells (killers/suppressors) is now recognised and the Th/Ts relationship is an important immunoregulatory index that plays an essential role in the maintenance of a normal immune response.

1011 (FA-315)	Fundamental aspects	GRP in SORP Pus lesions and RANACH.
Immune response - the potential of Treg cells?		

Evidence has been obtained that the immunosuppressive potential of Treg cells can be inhibited:

to be temporarily neutralised - due to the influence of a large amount of interleukin-2 (which is observed in the first stages of immune inflammation, which may be due to persistence of the inflammatory process)

blocked - through the production of interleukin-6 by antigen-presenting cells after their stimulation by microbial agents

The mechanisms of suppressive effects of Treg and Th3 include secretion of the inhibitory cytokines interleukin-10

Proof that Treg cells have an integrative role is the fact that they direct the immune response not only to auto-athigens, but also to foreign (and, above all, infectious) ones.

After activation by both auto- and foreign antigens, these cells acquire the necessary suppressive potential, which allows them to inhibit the proliferation of "naive" T lymphocytes.

A particularly important circumstance is that the concentration of antigens to activate the suppressive function of Treg-
cells is less than that required for T lymphocyte proliferation.

Thus, Treg cells:

on the one hand - control the development of tolerance (prevent the development of autoimmune processes)

on the other hand - regulate the immune response when a foreign agent enters the organism

It should be considered that a variety of factors influence the appearance of TIZ cells:

the Treg cells themselves

cytokines (interleukin-10, etc.) dexamethasone
vitamin D3
Treg cells inhibit in monocytes/macrophages the ability to produce pro-inflammatory cytokines.
It should be emphasised that among the various endogenous mechanisms of immunoregulation, the cytokine network occupies an important place, which ensures mutual communication between immunocompetent and other cells, which is mediated by molecules (receptors) that they actually produce (secretion, expression).
Each cytokine binds to its specific receptor on the surface of the target cell, and a cytokine activation signal is delivered inside the cell, which is transmitted to the cell nucleus and is usually realised through induction of expression of a particular gene or group of genes.

1012 (FA-316)	Fundamental aspects	GRP in SORP Pus lesions and RANACH.
Is the immune response a class of "cytokines"?		

Currently, more than 300 types of molecules are known that belong to the class of "cytokines" in the broad sense of the term (a major factor in intercellular communications); these are:
■=> interleukins
■=> monokines
■=> growth factors
■=> interferons
■=> tumour necrosis factor, etc.
However, even with regard to those cytokines, the pathogenetic role of which has been proved in purulent lesions (interleukins 1 and 6, interferon-gamma, tumour necrosis factor) and the functional purpose of which in the development of these diseases has been more or less clarified, it is still impossible to convincingly say that only due to some of them a certain function of certain cells is performed or disturbed.
Thus, macrophages produce tumour necrosis factor-alpha, which, in turn, causes expression of adhesive molecules on endothelial cells, which is necessary for migration of both neutrophils and macrophages themselves into the zone of bacterial damage. But, the same cytokine is also produced

by damaged epitheliocytes and activated endothelial cells. In general, tumour necrosis factor has multiple functions:

■=> affects the synthesis of interferons and opsonins

■=> activates all cells involved in the inflammatory-reparative process (and changes their phenotype).

■=> is an inducer of a sharp increase in the level of C-reactive protein in the blood in the acute phase of inflammation

■=> is a synergist of colony-stimulating factors that enhance proliferative processes

1013 (FA-317)	Fundamental aspects	GRP in SORP Pus lesions and RANACH.
The immune response - a role for interferon-gamma?		

The ability to "duplicate", synergistic functions is also characteristic of interferon-gamma, which:

On the one hand, it is a specialised inducer of macrophage activation (induces the expression of more than 100 different genes in the macrophage genome); however, activated T-lymphocytes and natural killer cells are also producers of this molecule.

■=> on the other hand - it induces and stimulates the production of other pro-inflammatory cytokines (tumour necrosis factor-alpha, interleukin-1, interleukin-6)

■=> In addition, it induces and stimulates the expression of class II histocompatibility antigens on macrophage membranes

■=> dramatically enhances effector (antimicrobial and antitumour) functions of macrophages by increasing the production of superoxide and nitroxide radicals by the cells

■=> enhances the expression of Fc receptors to immunoglobulin G and is thus an activator of immune phagocytosis and antibody-mediated cytotoxicity of macrophages themselves

The activating effect on macrophages is also mediated by the induction of their secretion of interferon-gamma itself, which affects the expression of macrophage receptors not only for antibodies but also for interferon-gamma .

dependent opsonisation, but also to the third complement fraction

1014 (FA-318)	Fundamental aspects	GRP in SORP and Wound Pus Injuries
The immune response - a common pattern?		

When analysing the overall immune response pattern, it is very important to consider the existence of not only Th1 and Th2, which provide different immune scenarios (cellular or humoral response), but also a set of regulatory cells (Treg, Th3) that:

- => direct the immune response
- => maintain immune homeostasis (homeostatic balance of the functioning of the immune system itself) by preventing it from reacting to its own (self) antigens
- => when responding to foreign antigens, in particular infectious antigens, they "stop" the development of the immune response at the necessary time and bring the immune system into a state of equilibrium.

A decrease in the number of regulatory cells can lead to the development of allergy. Thus, the study of the factors of intercellular relations, both at the organismal level and at the level of their relations with pathogens of purulent infections, can contribute to the development of new effective pathogenetically based methods of treatment of appropriate patients.

At the same time, the development of purulent processes would be impossible in case of incomplete functioning of natural and adaptive links of the immune response.

Despite the fact that, from a phylogenetic point of view, the antigen-nonspecific immune response is older than the antigen-specific immune response, their mechanisms remain incompletely understood. In addition, there are other factors and processes that enhance the above-mentioned parts of the immune system, such as the role of opsonisation factors, without which the immune response is practically impossible.

This realisation occurs directly through different types of molecules of intercellular relationships, in which primarily cytokines and adhesion molecules are important.

In antigen-specific (rapid, innate) immune response reactions, the detection of pathogens is based on the recognition of common molecules that signal the foreignness of their carriers.

In reactions of antigen-nonspecific (slow, acquired, adaptive) immune response, pathogen recognition is directed to individual molecules or their fragments that are specific only for a particular pathogen.
It is incorrect to give the role of the initiator of immunological changes to any one of the departments of the immune system, as they are both aimed at the elimination of the pathogenic factor and the restoration of immunological disorders created by it.
The function of "working together" is evolutionarily characteristic of the immune system, and it was formed in the same way during the evolution of the "microorganism-macroorganism" relationship.

1015 (FA-319)	Fundamental aspects	GRP in SORP and Wound Pus Injuries
Immune response - research findings?		

In patients with purulent-inflammatory lesions of superficial tissues various changes in cellular and molecular blood systems were revealed. Deviations from
physiological values of peripheral blood parameters were insignificant.
The study of NST-test recovery activity, which reflects the state of bactericidal peroxidase systems of cells and correlates with the formation of superoxide radicals, indicates a decrease in the level of general non-specific resistance of the organism:

- => the mean cytochemical ratio was reduced by an average of 1.3-fold
- => neutrophil activity reserve index - by 1.8 times
- => number of unstimulated neutrophils increased by 1.4 times
- => number of stimulated neutrophils - by 1.4 times

Determination of the ratios of lymphocyte differentiation clusters showed:

- => increase in the proportional content of lymphocytes with suppressive function in blood

(CD8) compared to the number of lymphocytes with helper function (CD4).

- => CD4/CD8 ratio was on average 0.8 (normal - 1.21.3)
- => there were certain changes in serum immunoglobulins in correlation with changes in lymphocytes

Adhesive molecules (ICAM-1) and interleukins 8 and 10, the levels of which were significantly elevated (2.7-, 4.5- and 7.5-fold, respectively), were examined in serum with additional factors of intercellular relations.

1016 (FA-320)	Fundamental aspects	GRP in SORP Pus lesions, and RANACH.
Immune response - a rationale for complex therapy?		

Taking into account the above-mentioned peculiarities of changes in the nonspecific and adaptive parts of the immune response, in the system of complex treatment of the corresponding patients we recommended the technique with the use of immunomodulator (ribomunil) and vitamin-mineral complex (miltrium with beta-carotene).

The vaccinating effect of bacterial ribosomes, which are included in ribomunil, is complemented by non-specific immune stimulation due to the presence of proteoglycans of the cell membrane of C. pneumoniae in the preparation; however, one of the most important points is that ribomunil causes the activation of specific antibodies, which determines the state of post-vaccine immunity.

Miltrium with beta-carotene potentiates the effects of ribomunil. With its 13 vitamins, it affects at least 20 different pathogenetic mechanisms that may occur in such lesions, and with its 16 trace elements it affects another 16 different metabolic mechanisms. This is why the main effects of its administration are:

- => reduce the risk of infectious diseases
- => increased immune defence response
- => improved metabolism
- => significant effects on the function of epithelial and endothelial cells, neurons
- => promotes tissue regeneration processes

The use of these two drugs in the system of complex therapy restores the disturbed indices of non-specific and adaptive immune response, and in this regard can be recommended for widespread implementation in practice.

1017 (FA-321)	Fundamental aspects	GRP in SORP and Wound Pus Injuries
The wound process - "concepts"?		

A wound process is:

■=> where body reactions, both local and general, occur in response to a wound for subsequent wound healing

■=> wound healing is characterised by clinical, bacteriological, biochemical, pathophysiological, structural changes (in the dynamics of the process)

■=> the above changes in response to damage are a complex set of biological reactions with its realisation at the local level

■=> local changes are characterised by consistency and are closely linked to multifaceted organism-wide reactions

1018 (FA-322)	Fundamental aspects	GRP in SORP and Wound Pus Injuries
Is the wound process a healing process?		

Wound healing is a manifestation of adaptation with a complex of complex biological processes in the wound defect that culminate in healing.

The distinctive features of this process are cyclicality and phasing (periods).

1019 (FA-323)	Fundamental aspects	GRP in SORP Pus lesions and RANACH.
Wound process - classifications?		

Analysing the available classifications of the wound process, we can conclude that to the greatest extent correspond to the dynamics of clinical manifestations those of them, which distinguish:

■=> the preparatory period, which determines the course of action subsequent changes (inflammatory phase)
■=> basic processes of wound tissue repair (proliferation/regeneration phase)
■=> reorganisation phase (maturation and scar formation)

1020 (FA-324)	Fundamental aspects	GRP in SORP Pus lesions and RANACH.
The wound process - reactions?		

The reactions of the organism to a wound (trauma) are characterised by stages:

- ■ => vasospasm in the wound area (initial reaction)
- ■ => vasodilation (replaces spasm)
- ■ => increased permeability of the vascular wall
- ■ => traumatic oedema - fast-onset.
- ■ => tissue alteration (localised)
- ■ => metabolic disorder (local):
  - o acidosis
  - o hyperosmia
  - o colloidal changes
  - o others
- ■ => increasing oedema:
  - o narrows the wound canal (until it disappears)
  - o dead blood-soaked canal tissues are squeezed out (so-called "primary wound cleansing")

■=> histamine and serotonin, released when blood vessels dilate, further in turn:

- o dilate arterioles and venules
- o accelerate capillary blood flow
- o increase capillary permeability
- o stimulate phagocytosis
- o speed up the bleeding time

1021 (FA-325)	Fundamental aspects	GRP in SORP Pus lesions and RANACH.
Wound process - exudate (general information)?		

The exudate formed as a result of increased vascular permeability and release of water and blood formations in the first 2-3 days contains polymorphonuclear leukocytes to a greater extent, later mononuclear cells (lymphocytes, monocytes/macrophages).

1022 (FA-326)	Fundamental aspects	GRP in SORP and Wound Pus Injuries
Is the wound process an exudate (neutrophils)?		

The main role of neutrophils in exudate is that they:

- => to a greater extent - phagocytise the microorganism
- => phagocytise necrotic tissue to a lesser extent
- => lysate non-viable elements
- => secrete inflammatory mediators

In their specific granules, neutrophils contain substances (e.g. lactoferrin) that deaden phagocytised microorganisms.

Non-specific granules (azurophilic) contain biological substances (lysozyme, etc.) that are necessary for intracellular proteolysis to clear the wound of necrotised masses.

A major role is played by cathepsins, which can not only degrade kininogens, but also modify already secreted kinins. The function of lysis of altered collagen fibres in the foci of destruction is also important.

But neutrophils themselves, after performing their functions, decay and are phagocytised by macrophages, which, in addition, also phagocytise necrotic tissues destroyed by neutrophils, products of bactericidal decay (the process of wound cleansing).

1023 (FA-327)	Fundamental aspects	GRP in SORP and Wound Pus Injuries
Is the wound process an exudate (lymphocytes)?		

The role of lymphocytes in purulent inflammation is complex:

■=> they are the source of plasma cells (synthesising antibodies)

■=> enhance or support fibroblast growth (through the mechanism of genetic information transfer)

1024 (FA-328)	Fundamental aspects	GRP in SORP Pus lesions and RANACH.
Is the wound process an exudate (microbial flora)?		

The role of microbial flora in purulent inflammation is complex:

■=> promotes inflammation

■=> involved in proteolysis of dead tissue

■=> may have a negative impact on the wound process (wound contamination)

■=> it is an indispensable participant in wound healing

1025 (FA-329)	Fundamental aspects	GRP in SORP and Wound Pus Injuries
Is the wound process an inflammatory response?		

In the wound process, the inflammatory response proceeds in stages and is characterised by:

■=> rapidity - a leucocytic wall is formed at the border of dead and viable tissues (already on the first day)

■=> the phase of granulation tissue development (filling the wound defect) starts on the 3-4th day:

- o white blood cells are getting smaller
- o macrophages - persist

o fibroblasts and capillary endothelial cells - play a major role in proliferation

1026 (FA-330)	Fundamental aspects	GRP in SORP Pus lesions and RANACH.
Is the wound process scarring?		

Collagen produced by fibroblasts is of the greatest importance in wound scarring, and collagen binding occurs with the participation of DNA synthesised by them, the new formation of neutral mucopolysaccharides and acidic glycosaminoglycans.

In the granulation tissue, glycosaminoglycans form the basis of the interstitial substance, and after 6-7 days antibody-producing plasma cells are also found in it.

On the 12th-30th day, the final phase of the scarring process occurs:

■=> the number of cellular elements and microvessels progressively decreases

■=> both collagen fibre formation and partial collagen fibre destruction take place in parallel

■=> fine regulation of processes - both fibrotic tissue formation and scar tissue accumulation and resorption - is carried out

1027 (FA-331)	Fundamental aspects	GRP in SORP Pus Infections and RANACH.
Is the wound process a contraction?		

Wound contraction (uniform concentric contraction of the wound edges and walls) reflects the balance between the formation and resorption of granulation and scar tissue. This process combines in different phases of wound healing:

■=> with intensive epithelialisation (starts with the formation of argyrophilic fibres)

■=> with gradual pushing of the epithelium over the wound edges with partial destruction of the epithelium

■=> with further epithelial overgrowth of the mature granulation tissue and its differentiation

1028 (FA-332)	Fundamental aspects	GRP in SORP Pus Infections and RANACH.
Wound process - regeneration (general information)?		

Regarding general information on wound regeneration, it should be

to note the following:

■=> on the one hand, it is the renewal of the structures of the organism in the process of life activity

■=> on the other hand, it is the restoration of structures that are lost as a result of pathological processes

■=> this mechanism is deployed at different levels of the organism:

- systemic
- organ
- tissue
- cellular
- intracellular

■=> the basis of the process is the pronounced ability of epithelium (including SORPs) to proliferate, due to their basic function - continuous maintenance of tissue integrity at the boundary with the environment

1029 (FA-333)	Fundamental aspects	GRP in SORP Pus Infections and RANACH.
Wound process - regeneration (forms)?		

The forms of regeneration (cellular and intracellular) are based on a single phenomenon - HYPERPLASION OF NUCLEAR AND CYTOPLASMATIC STRUCTURES.

1030 (FA-334)	Fundamental aspects	GRP in SORP Pus Infections and RANACH.

Wound process - regeneration (common distinguishing features)?

The general distinctive features of wound healing (regenerative process) can be traced back to the so-called removed skin flap, where a scar is formed that differs in structure from the excised area.

In the area surrounding the wound, after tightening of the edges, hyperplasia and hypertrophy of cells occur, the task of which is to provide the lost mass. In cases of atypical regeneration, the regenerated tissue differs significantly from the lost tissue both in structure and shape.

Thus, SORP regeneration (by analogy with skin) differs from that in internal organs, as 4 consecutive processes occur during it:

- => wound contraction (tightening of the defect edges)
- => insertion growth (outside the wound)
- => formation of new tissue (in the defect)
- => transformation of new tissue into a complex of immature cells (regenerate) in the area of injury

1031 (FA-335)	Fundamental aspects	GRP in SORP Pus Infections and RANACH.
Is the wound process regeneration (edge tightening)?		

The process of tightening the wound edges is characterised by the following:

- => is concentric in nature
- => it's a compensatory process
- => the area of damage includes undamaged tissue together with its specific structures

1032 (FA-336)	Fundamental aspects	GRP in SORP Pus Infections and RANACH.
Wound process - regeneration (out of wound growth)?		

Insertional growth (outside the wound) is:
∎=> the process of overgrowth of damaged tissue elements around the wound, aimed at replenishing them
∎=> it is a response to the duration of the contracting processes
∎=> the area of the defect is a defined gap of compensatory response
∎=> increased mitotic activity of the epithelium
persists after completion of wound epithelialisation

1033 (FA-337)	Fundamental aspects	GRP in SORP Pus Infections and RANACH.
Is the wound process regeneration ("regenerate")?		

The regenerate that forms at the site of the defect may retain specific structures of previously intact tissue, and it :
∎=> formed - long term
∎=> continues - and after epithelialisation of the defect
∎=> formed - always atypical and incomplete

1034 (FA-338)	Fundamental aspects	GRP in SORP Pus Infections and RANACH.
Is the wound process regeneration (young tissue)?		

In young tissues:
∎=> all specific structures are laid down, and this occurs in different phases of the regenerative process
∎=> impossible to realign
a connective tissue scar at the site of the defect and the epithelium that covers it
∎=> consists mainly of thick collagen bundles
fibres

1035 (FA-339)	Fundamental aspects	GRP in SORP Pus Infections and RANACH.
Is the wound process regeneration (deficient collagen)?		

Fibrillogenesis leads to the incompleteness of collagen, which is easily degenerated. In scars, the transition of some fibroblasts into fibrocytes is delayed. These processes can be influenced by hormones that reduce the mitotic activity of proliferating epithelium by:

■=> suppression - development of inflammatory oedema
■=> suppression of phagocytic activity of macrophages
■=> restrictions - granulation tissue development

1036 (FA-340)	Fundamental aspects	GRP in SORP and Wound Pus Injuries
Wound process - regeneration (influence of hormones)?		

Data on the effects of hormones on regeneration are conflicting, but with regard to sex hormones, most scientists emphasise their positive effects on wound healing.

1037 (FA-341)	Fundamental aspects	GRP in SORP Pus lesions and RANACH.
Wound process - regeneration (influence of vitamin C)?		

Wound healing is slowed down by vitamin C deficiency, and it primarily depends on such causes:

■=> dramatic decrease in phosphatase activity in fibroblasts
■=> cessation of collagen synthesis by fibroblasts (fatty degeneration)

1038 (FA-342)	Fundamental aspects	GRP in SORP Pus Infections and RANACH.
Wound process - stages of development (inflammation)?		

From the 3 stages of purulent wound development to the stage of inflammation (the first one) already on the 3rd-7th day a number of processes (biochemical, pathophysiological) are observed, which influence the nature of subsequent events.

These processes largely depend on the microbiota in the wound - with the content in 1 cm^3 more than 100 thousand microbial bodies can occur generalisation of the process, up to wound sepsis.

The wound process in dentistry is frequently observed, but it is when pathogenic microbiota invade the wound that a purulent wound is formed, especially when the body's resistance is insufficient, both in general and in the area of damaged tissues.

Wound healing by primary tension in case of massive microbial contamination becomes impossible. This distinguishes purulent wounds non-specific (putrefactive, etc.) and specific (diphtheria, etc.).

1039 (FA-343)	Fundamental aspects	GRP in SORP Pus lesions and RANACH.
Wound process - stages of development (regeneration)?		

In the second stage of wound healing (regeneration) a significant role belongs to fibroblasts - covering a thin layer of capillary loop, they prevent the penetration into the wound, both the microbes themselves and their toxins, as a result of which vascular disorders, oedema and intoxication are reduced .

1040 (FA-344)	Fundamental aspects	GRP in SORP Pus lesions and RANACH.

Wound process - stages of development (scar reorganisation)?

In the third stage (scar reorganisation), colloid formation occurs, which also depends on the abundance of fibroblasts in the granulation tissue.

1041 (FA-345)	Fundamental aspects	GRP in SORP Pus lesions and RANACH.
The wound process - general principles of management of purulent wounds?		

The detailed treatment of purulent wounds will be dealt with in the following volumes in relation to private dentistry. Here, however, we will only mention general principles based on the objectives of this volume (Fundamental Aspects of Dentistry). For the topical medication of purulent wounds, the principles are followed depending on the phase of the process.
In the first phase, the aim is to achieve at least 3 treatment effects:

- => suppression of infection
- => evacuation of contents
- => rejection of destroyed tissue

Antiseptics are used to suppress infection ,
multi-component ointments with a water-soluble base.
Hypertonic solutions and drainage are used to evacuate the contents; proteolytic enzymes are also used to remove dead tissue.
In the second phase, the aim is not only to suppress the infection, but also the growth of granulation. Therefore, in addition to ointments with chemopreventive agents and antiseptics, indifferent ointments such as Combutech, Algipore, etc. are used.

In the third phase, the aim is to epithelialise the wound and organise the scar, therefore, in addition to the above, ointments such as solcoseril etc. are also used.

As with the pathophysiological phases of development in relation to the clinical stages of a suppurative wound, appropriate principles are followed:

■=> into the first stage:

o suppression of microflora (including general antibiotic therapy)

o stimulation of the immune system

o removal of exudate and necrotised tissue

o improvement of tissue trophism and stimulation of anabolic processes (vitamin therapy, biostimulants)

o restoration of blood circulation at the site of injury (trental, sermion, etc.)

o use of proteolytic enzymes to increase membrane permeability to antibacterial agents, achieve anticoagulation, inhibit collagenase

■=> into stage two:

o preventing damage to granulation in the wound

o stimulation of granulation growth and wound epithelialisation o prevention of keloid development

■=> into stage three:

o keloid scar resorption (Phoebes, aloe, vitreous; physiotherapy, steroids)

In briefly summarising the principles of GRP development directly in the SORP to the dental practitioner, important points such as these should be reiterated:

• The surface area of the SORP is quite large, which favours colonisation and invasion of microorganisms

• This is due to the location under its epithelium of immune system cells capable of producing secretory immunoglobulin A

• The presence of the epithelial barrier prevents antigens from reaching the immune cells beneath it, and therefore they must:

about getting through the barrier

about being processed

o be presented to the cells of the immune system

The first visible stage of acute inflammation is haemodynamic changes, but vasodilatation is only a part of it, because local injection of vasodilators does not cause inflammation by itself; increased vascular permeability and accumulation of leukocytes in combination with chemoattractants of neutrophils (including those of microbial origin) are the most important moments of the subsequent stages of inflammatory reaction, when local extravasal accumulations appear at the sites of damage, infection, antigen-stimulation:

- leucocytes
- mesenchymal cells
- plasma proteins
- liquids

Thus, it is an integral part of the body's defence, preventing further damage.

In SORP, as a barrier (one of the factors of natural resistance) an important role (including anti-inflammatory) is played:

- secretion secreted by the mucocellular apparatus of the salivary glands (containing lysozyme)
- Microbial antagonism (associated with the presence of normal microbiota) - thus inhibiting a number of potentially pathogenic microorganisms

CHAPTER 4

Inflammatory-reparative process - nociceptive disorders in dental diseases

Nociceptive disorders in dental diseases

At the same time, the predominant complaint of dental patients is pain or other nociceptive sensations of the oral cavity structures (recall that they are the most important characteristic of the inflammatory pentad of Celsus-Galen). However, pain can also be of non-inflammatory nature - tumours, scar stretching, etc.

Since pain will be discussed in detail in subsequent volumes in specific pathological conditions, we will analyse in this volume only some of its fundamental aspects, as well as other nociceptive sensations that can be observed in the inflammatory-reparative process of SORP.

1042 (FA-346)	Fundamental aspects	HRP in STOMATOLOGICAL DEVELOPMENTS (nociception-antinociception)
The relevance of the problem of pain?		

The relevance of the problem of pain (including in dentistry) is due to the fact that relieving a person of this suffering is the most important task of a doctor (as well as his first duty - to save the life of the patient).

When this distressing sensation is chronicled, there is disorganisation of functional systems of the organism, psychophysiological state and behavioural reactions change.

However, unlike other sense modalities) is a special function that warns of danger, although it is simultaneous:

- protective
- has adaptive traits
- contains pathological manifestations

A number of dental diseases are not accompanied by pain sensations (periodontitis, caries), at the same time such categories of pain as neuropathic and terminal pain cause significant disintegration of the integral regulating neuroendocrine-immune system of the organism with the subsequent development of various pathological conditions.

1043 (FA-347)	Fundamental aspects	HRP in STOMATOLOGICAL DEVELOPMENTS (nociception-antinociception)
"Shades" of pain (terminology)?		

Terminological aspects of pain will be discussed in detail in the questions of its categories and classifications, but in scientific literature more than 100 shades of this burdensome sensation are described.

1044 (FA-348)	Fundamental aspects	HRP in STOMATOLOGICAL DEVELOPMENTS (nociception-antinociception)
Methods of dealing with pain?		

The problem of pain management is constantly attracting the attention of researchers, and many methods of pain control have been proposed, but:
There is no universal analgesic method (as there is no unified pathophysiological concept of pain).

1045 (FA-349)	Fundamental aspects	HRP in STOMATOLOGICAL DEVELOPMENTS (nociception-antinociception)
A conceptual understanding of pain?		

Why is the conceptual understanding of pain changing? It depends on the latest discoveries in neuroanatomy, neurophysiology, neuropharmacology, and human behavioural sciences.

1046 (FA-350)	Fundamental aspects	HRP in STOMATOLOGICAL DEVELOPMENTS (nociception-antinociception)
Nociceptive impulses?		

Two main issues remain problematic with regard to nociceptive impulsation:

- when such impulses cease to have physiological significance?
- when it becomes pain?

This is the reason why the question of how pain is managed by the various methods (pharmacological and non-pharmacological) is still problematic.

1047 (FA-351)	Fundamental aspects	HRP in STOMATOLOGICAL DEVELOPMENTS (nociception-antinociception)
Pain syndrome?		

In most nosological dental forms, pain is the most frequent or only symptom! Relieving or eliminating pain is one of the main tasks of dentistry.

1048 (FA-352)	Fundamental aspects	HRP in STOMATOLOGICAL DEVELOPMENTS (nociception-antinociception)
Dental manipulation and pain?		

Dental manipulations (diagnostic, treatment) may be accompanied by pain. At the same time, the view that pain intensity can be used as a criterion of treatment adequacy is erroneous.

1049 (FA-353)	Fundamental aspects	HRP in STOMATOLOGICAL DEVELOPMENTS (nociception-antinociception)
Adequacy of anaesthesia?		

Adequacy of anaesthesia provides:

- painless dental manipulations
- normal psychophysiological state of the patient
- drug tolerance

1050 (FA-354)	Fundamental aspects	HRP in STOMATOLOGICAL DEVELOPMENTS (nociception-antinociception)
The "concept" of pain?		

Although the notion of pain as nociception is considered the most logical, it is still substantiated mainly experimentally, but clinically all pain syndromes are complex concepts and therefore, relevant research should be extended in a fundamental aspect.

1051 (FA-355)	Fundamental aspects	HRP in STOMATOLOGICAL DEVELOPMENTS (nociception-antinociception)
Pain as an integrative function?		

In pain, many functional systems of the body are switched on, resulting in an integrative response involving:

- consciousnesses
- memories
- emotions
- autonomic response
- somatic response
- behavioural response

1052 (FA-356)	Fundamental aspects	HRP in STOMATOLOGICAL DEVELOPMENTS (nociception-antinociception)
Is pain an evolutionary process?		

Pain, as a type process, is evolutionarily developed in the organism, and such a reaction occurs both when nociceptive factors are acted upon and when antinociceptive systems are weakened.

1053 (FA-357)	Fundamental aspects	HRP in STOMATOLOGICAL DEVELOPMENTS (nociception-antinociception)

Classifications of pain?

Many classifications of pain have been proposed.

According to the classification of R. Schmidt (1985), according to the CHARACTER and LOCALISATION there are different:

- visceral pain (in the internal organs)
- somatic deep pain
  - bones
  - joints
  - connective tissue
  - muscles
- somatic superficial pain (skin, SORP) primary:
  - realised quickly
  - localised easily
  - when the stimulus is removed, it disappears
- superficial secondary:
  - realised slowly
  - it is poorly localised
  - lasts for a long time
  - has an unpleasant colour

Practical clinical classification distinguishes between these types of pain:

- spicy
- terminal
- neuropathic
- chronic
- psychogenic

The classification characterisation of pain also includes:

- Duration:
  - up to 4 weeks - acute

4-12 weeks - subacute

- more than 12 weeks - chronic
- localisation of the irritation/damage:

about nociceptors - nocigenic pain

about the peripheral or central nervous system

- neurogenic pain

1054 (FA-358)	Fundamental aspects	HRP in STOMATOLOGICAL DEVELOPMENTS (nociception-antinociception)
Pain - as a symptom?		

Not only in inflammation, but also in other pathologies, pain is most often one of the symptoms - an unpleasant sensory and emotional experience related to existing or potential tissue damage, or - described in terms of such damage.

1055 (FA-359)	Fundamental aspects	HRP in STOMATOLOGICAL DEVELOPMENTS (nociception-antinociception)
Algogens?		

Algogens are factors that cause the sensation of pain (nociceptive); of these:

exogenous include:

- mechanical:
  - compression
  - section
  - stretching
  - bump
  - others
- physical:
  - light
  - sound
  - temperature (high, low)
  - barometric pressure (high, low)
  - others

- chemical:
- o alkalis
- o acids
- o salt
- o others

the endogenous ones include:

- substance P
- kinins
- prostaglandins
- histamine
- acetylcholine
- others

Various nociceptors respond to stimuli:

- myelinated (high threshold)
- o small receptive fields
- o signal conduction velocity 20t m/s
- o respond to mechanical stimuli
- unmyelinated (polymodal):
- o sufficiently large receptive fields
- o signal conduction speed 0.5-2 m/s
- o react to mechanical stimuli, as well as to chemical and thermal stimuli

Algogens accumulate as a result of tissue damage, which leads to increased sensitivity of nociceptors at the site of damage (spontaneous activity, decreased excitation threshold), and to further sensitisation of nociceptors:

- hyperalgesia - a pronounced pain sensation at the mild painful irritation
- allodynia - pain sensation with non-painful stimuli

Pain is subjected to different types of treatments:

- sensory-discriminatory (assessing the quality, strength, duration of pain impact)
- affective-motivational (the need to avoid pain is formed)
- evaluative-cognitive (provided by the level of attention , anxiety, memory, experience, auditory and visual participation)

It is important to note that all qualitative characteristics of pain sensation are genetically determined and are generated in the brain, with peripheral stimuli being only non-specific triggers.

1056 (FA-360)	Fundamental aspects	HRP in STOMATOLOGICAL DEVELOPMENTS (nociception-antinociception)
Role of the antinociceptive system (general information)?		

Pain can also be caused by abnormalities in the antinociceptive system:

- serotonergic
- noradrenergic
- GABAergic
- opioidergic:

o beta-endorphin o meth-enkephalin o leu-enkephalin o dynorphin

1057 (FA-361)	Fundamental aspects	HRP in STOMATOLOGICAL DEVELOPMENTS (nociception-antinociception)
The role of information correlation?		

Violation of the relationship between pain and other afferent information (coming from other types of receptors - tactile, proprioreceptors, etc.) may also be one of the causes of pain syndrome.

1058 (FA-362)	Fundamental aspects	HRP in STOMATOLOGICAL DEVELOPMENTS (nociception-antinociception)
Pain as a reflex process?		

As a reflex process, pain involves all the main links of the reflex arc:
■=> receptors
■=> pulse conductors
■=> mediators
■=> formations of the brain (spinal cord and brain)

1059 (FA-363)	Fundamental aspects	HRP in STOMATOLOGICAL DEVELOPMENTS (nociception-antinociception)
Specificity theory (Frey)?		

Frey's theory of specificity is the first scientifically based theory of the essence of pain, and according to its tenets, the presence of e is recognised:
■=> specific pain nociceptors
■=> specific afferent pain pathways

1060 (FA-364)	Fundamental aspects	HRP in STOMATOLOGICAL DEVELOPMENTS (nociception-antinociception)
Intensity theory (Goldstader)?		

According to Goldstadter's intensity theory, the presence of special pain receptors is not recognised and the leading importance is given to the intensity of the stimulus, in particular when low-threshold mechano- and thermoreceptors are affected by stimuli with an intensity that exceeds a critical level.

1061 (FA-365)	Fundamental aspects	HRP in STOMATOLOGICAL DEVELOPMENTS (nociception-antinociception)
Is the theory "unifying" (Revenko)?		

This theory recognises that there are specialised nociceptive neurons with C-axons:

■=> low-frequency (less than 2 Hz) exposures they are aroused by non-painful stimuli

■=> high-frequency (over 2 Hz) they are excited by painful stimuli

1062 (FA-366)	Fundamental aspects	HRP in STOMATOLOGICAL DEVELOPMENTS (nociception-antinociception)
Pattern theory (Weddel)?		

According to pattern theory, all types of sensitivity are the result of spatial and temporal patterns of impulses, and when nonspecific receptors are strongly stimulated, a pattern typical of pain is produced.

1063 (FA-367)	Fundamental aspects	HRP in STOMATOLOGICAL DEVELOPMENTS (nociception-antinociception)
Properties of nociceptors?		

Nociceptors are characterised by:

■=> these are high-threshold formations

■=> their arousal threshold is variable

■=> the value of the sensitivity threshold depends on the receptor localisation

1064 (FA-368)	Fundamental aspects	HRP in STOMATOLOGICAL DEVELOPMENTS (nociception-antinociception)
Nociceptors of the pulp?		

Pulp nociceptors have a low threshold of sensitivity (as do skin, external genitalia, periosteum).

1065 (FA-369)	Fundamental aspects	HRP in STOMATOLOGICAL DEVELOPMENTS (nociception-antinociception)
Mechanism of excitation of pain receptors?		

Under the action of algogens, the membrane permeability of pain receptors increases, which is the cause (mechanism) of their excitation.

1066 (FA-370)	Fundamental aspects	HRP in STOMATOLOGICAL DEVELOPMENTS (nociception-antinociception)
The role of interconnections of nervous system formations?		

Three interconnected entities of the nervous system (conductors, subcortical and cortical structures of the brain) are involved not only in the transmission but also in the formation of pain sensations.

There are certain differences with respect to the conduction of impulses by the fibres:

■ => A-delta fibres - responsible for the formation of so-called "primary" pain (impulse velocity of 4-30 m/s)

■ => C-fibres - form "secondary" pain (impulse conduction velocity - 0.4-2.0 m/s)

■ => primary pain fibres terminate in the nucleus cerebri of the trigeminal pathway and at the base of the posterior horns of the spinal cord; the function of this spinothalamic pathway is to transmit pain and temperature sensitivity signals

■ => except for the spinothalamic pathway (first neuron

The lemniscus system (represented by thick fibres), hypothalamus, reticular formation, limbic system, somatosensory zone of the cerebral cortex are also important in the formation of pain.

1067 (FA-371)	Fundamental aspects	HRP in STOMATOLOGICAL DEVELOPMENTS (nociception-antinociception)
Pain mediators - different mechanisms of action?		

Pain mediators involved in its formation, pain conduction and intensity control have certain differences at different levels of the nervous system:

■ => they have an excitatory effect at the receptor level:

- histamine
- prostaglandins
- serotonin
- acetylcholine

■ => enhances conduction of impulses at the level of primary afferents - substance P; inhibit: noradrenaline, GABA, glycine, neurotensin, cholecystokinin

■ => serotonin has both enhancing and inhibitory effects

■ => at the level of the posterior horns of the spinal cord increase the conduction of impulses:

- glutamate
- Substance P

- cholecystokinin
- neurotensin

inhibit: o enkephalin o acetylcholine o GABA

- serotonin
- dopamine
- noradrenaline

Thus, some mediators can act at different levels of the nervous system (serotonin, GABA, substance P, and others).

1068 (FA-372)	Fundamental aspects	HRP in STOMATOLOGICAL DEVELOPMENTS (nociception-antinociception)
Structures of the antinociceptive system?		

The structures of the antinociceptive system have their own distinctive mechanisms (morphological, biochemical, physical), and their functioning requires a constant inflow of afferent information.

The controlling elements of this system are represented by:

- at the segmental level
- at centre levels
- by humoral mechanisms

1069 (FA-373)	Fundamental aspects	HRP in STOMATOLOGICAL DEVELOPMENTS (nociception-antinociception)
Mechanisms of opiate analgesia - general information?		

Adding to what was previously said about opiates, it should be reemphasised that these compounds (enkephalins and endorphins) are formed by the breakdown of a common source (the pituitary hormone beta-lipotropin).

Endorphins are more localised and are contained mainly in the hypothalamus, while they are released into blood plasma and spinal fluid only when necessary, and then contact their receptors located at different levels of the nociceptive system (including peripheral receptors).
Enkephalins are more widely localised in the CNS:

- in the posterior horns of the spinal cord
- in the reticular formation
- in the hypothalamic nuclei
- in the frontal cortex of the large cerebral hemispheres.

Unlike endorphins, they do not bind to their receptors through the blood or liquor, but directly (locally).

1070 (FA-374)	Fundamental aspects	HRP in STOMATOLOGICAL DEVELOPMENTS (nociception-antinociception)
Are the mechanisms of analgesia adrenergic?		

Adrenergic mechanisms of anaesthesia are realised by norepinephrine, dopamine and serotonin. With the help of noradrenaline:

- inhibits the conduction of pain impulses at the level of the spinal cord, brainstem and reticular formation
- Activation of central adrenergic structures and formation of analgesia with suppression of emotional-behavioural and hemodynamic manifestations under strong pain influence
- activation of the sympathoadrenal system and mobilisation of tropic hormones occurs when a stress response is applied

1071 (FA-375)	Fundamental aspects	HRP in STOMATOLOGICAL DEVELOPMENTS (nociception-antinociception)

Mechanisms of pain relief - other hormone products?

100-1000 times stronger than the ecephalins have an analgesic effect:
■=> vasopressin
■=> angiotensin
■=> oxytocin
■=> somatostatin ■=> neurotensin

1072 (FA-376)	Fundamental aspects	HRP in STOMATOLOGICAL DEVELOPMENTS (nociception-antinociception)
Are the mechanisms of analgesia serotonergic?		

Evidence of the serotoninergic system's involvement in analgesia (indirect !) is the phenomenon of serotonin headache, before the onset of which vasoconstriction is observed as a result of excess serotonin in the blood plasma. Serotonin is subsequently excreted in the urine (in an altered form) and broken down. After that, its level also decreases in brain structures.

1073 (FA-377)	Fundamental aspects	HRP in STOMATOLOGICAL DEVELOPMENTS (nociception-antinociception)
Are the mechanisms of analgesia cholinergic?		

The accumulation of acetylcholine activates the cholinergic system and thus enhances morphine analgesia. It is also possible that acetylcholine stimulates the release of opioid peptides by binding to M - cholinoreceptors.

1074 (FA-378)	Fundamental aspects	HRP in STOMATOLOGICAL DEVELOPMENTS (nociception-antinociception)
Are the mechanisms of analgesia GABAergic?		

Gamma-aminobutyric acid (GABA) inhibits emotional and behavioural responses to pain and thus adaptation to pain stress is ensured.

GABA-positive drugs (baclofen, depakine) potentiate the effects of narcotic analgesics.

1075 (FA-379)	Fundamental aspects	HRP in STOMATOLOGICAL DEVELOPMENTS (nociception-antinociception)
Categories of pain - general information?		

In dental practice, the major clinical categories of pain include:

■=> acute

■=> post-operative

■=> neuropathic

■=> terminal

■=> chronic

■=> psychogenic

1076 (FA-380)	Fundamental aspects	HRP in STOMATOLOGICAL DEVELOPMENTS (nociception-antinociception)

Categories of pain - acute (causes of onset)?

The causes of acute pain are:

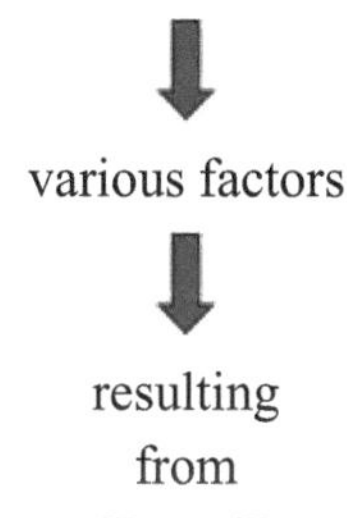

various factors

resulting from

trauma and pathological process

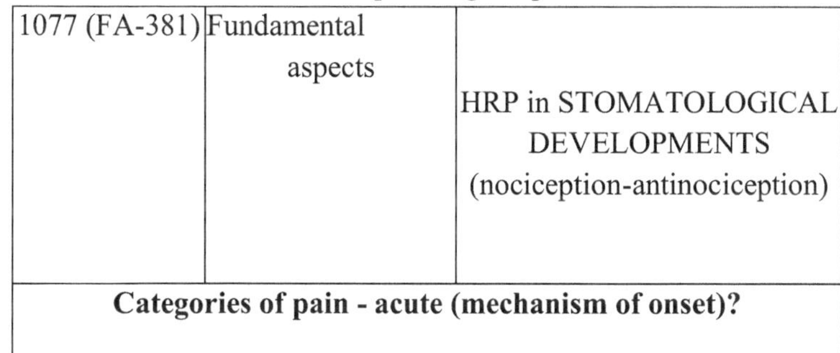

1077 (FA-381)	Fundamental aspects	HRP in STOMATOLOGICAL DEVELOPMENTS (nociception-antinociception)

Categories of pain - acute (mechanism of onset)?

One of the mechanisms of acute pain is excitation of nociceptors:

■=> this leads to the formation of electron pulses

■=> impulses along the conductive pathways reach the cortex cerebrum

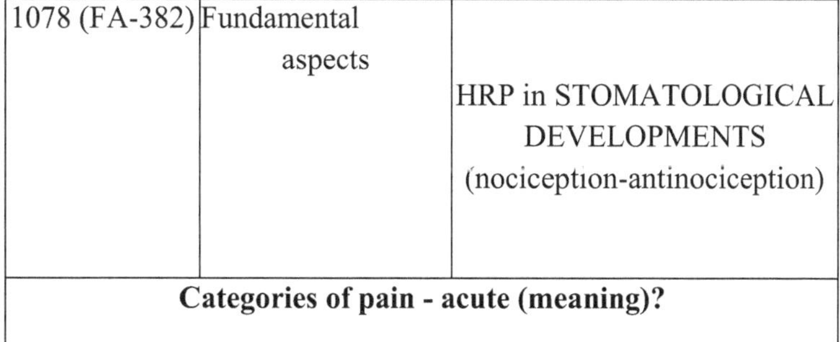

1078 (FA-382)	Fundamental aspects	HRP in STOMATOLOGICAL DEVELOPMENTS (nociception-antinociception)

Categories of pain - acute (meaning)?

The significance of acute pain in its biological utility:

■=> prevents threatening tissue damage

■=> it's one of the stress response factors

1079 (FA-383)	Fundamental aspects	HRP in STOMATOLOGICAL DEVELOPMENTS (nociception - antinociception)
Categories of pain - acute (features)?		

The features of acute pain are:
waiting for pain to occur or disappear
increased pain perception with anxiety
self-restraint

1080 (FA-384)	Fundamental aspects	HRP in STOMATOLOGICAL DEVELOPMENTS (nociception - antinociception)
Categories of pain - acute (effective interventions)?		

Pathogenetically based effective interventions for acute pain are:
Non-steroidal and steroidal anti-inflammatory drugs
local anaesthetics
anxiolytics
narcotic analgesics
Psychological methods can only be of little help.

1081 (FA-385)	Fundamental aspects	HRP in STOMATOLOGICAL DEVELOPMENTS (nociception-antinociception)
Categories of pain - acute (pulpitis - pathogenesis)?		

The pain syndrome in pulpitis is a striking example of acute pain.

Pathogenetic causes in its occurrence are:
alteration of pulp components
effects of isolated biologically active substances
exudate exposure
pulp hypoxia
acidosis
decreased phagocyte activity

1082 (FA-386)	Fundamental aspects	HRP in STOMATOLOGICAL DEVELOPMENTS (nociception-antinociception)
Categories of pain - acute (pulpitis - a feature of inflammation)?		

The inflammatory reaction in pulpitis has its own peculiarities:
the space in which the oedema develops

- closed
- surrounded by bone hard tissue or dentin

any increase in pressure in the pulp chamber is accompanied by a pronounced pain syndrome
metabolic shifts can exacerbate pain

1083 (FA-387)	Fundamental aspects	HRP in STOMATOLOGICAL DEVELOPMENTS (nociception-antinociception)
Categories of pain - acute (pulpitis - pathogenetic treatment)?		

Taking into account the pathogenetic features of pulpitis, it is advisable to prescribe drugs that inhibit the synthesis of biologically active substances that lead to the development of inflammation at the site of lesion (prostaglandins, etc.).

The use of drugs that block the conduction of impulses along the nerve trunk is ineffective, as pain in pulpitis irradiates along the branches of the trigeminal nerve - from receptors in the nerve endings of the pulp along the maxillary and mandibular nerves, and along the spinothalamic pathway pain impulses reach the corresponding areas of the cortex of the cerebral hemispheres.

1084 (FA-388)	Fundamental aspects	HRP in STOMATOLOGICAL DEVELOPMENTS (nociception-antinociception)
Categories of pain - postoperative (general information)?		

The peculiarities of postoperative pain are that it consists of:
"wound" pain (from the area of the injury)
headache
worries
nausea may occur with some types of it,
vomiting, etc.

1085 (FA-389)	Fundamental aspects	HRP in STOMATOLOGICAL DEVELOPMENTS (nociception-antinociception)
Categories of pain - postoperative (autonomous reactions)?		

With postoperative pain, so-called "autonomic reactions" may develop, which can lead to complications and prevent the performance of necessary procedures (in particular - physiotherapy).

1086 (FA-390)	Fundamental aspects	HRP in STOMATOLOGICAL DEVELOPMENTS (nociception-antinociception)
Categories of pain - postoperative (mechanisms of development)?		

The mechanisms of development in such pain are:

damage to various tissue structures

activation of cutaneous and muscular afferentations (as a result of cutting and traction)

Further on, muscle soreness (as a result of its persistent reflex spasm) plays a role.

Thus, it is possible to note a combination of mechanisms of postoperative pain formation.

1087 (FA-391)	Fundamental aspects	HRP in STOMATOLOGICAL DEVELOPMENTS (nociception-antinociception)
Categories of pain - postoperative (pathogenetic treatment)?		

Reducing the influence of the various components of postoperative pain and managing factors that may increase the response to it (anxiety, depression) are the main areas of treatment of such pain syndrome. Should be carried out:

nociceptor blockade (topical)

Conductive blockade (with local anaesthetics)

spinal blockade

anti-inflammatory therapy

central antinociception (if necessary)

1088 (FA-392)	Fundamental aspects	HRP in STOMATOLOGICAL DEVELOPMENTS (nociception-antinociception)
Categories of pain - neuropathic (general information)?		

Among the common characteristics of neuropathic pain are:
lack of biological feasibility
Lack of a clear definition of neurological damage
understudied mechanisms:
nociceptive
conductive
sensory-anatomical deficits
inhibitions
adverse psychological effects

1089 (FA-393)	Fundamental aspects	HRP in STOMATOLOGICAL DEVELOPMENTS (nociception-antinociception)
Categories of pain - neuropathic (pain induction)?		

The development of so-called "pain induction" in peripheral nerve injury may play a role:
nerve dysfunction - "pain triggering".
generation of ectopic impulses by mechanically sensitive nerves
"cross-talk" between nerve fibres (small and large)
shifts in information processing (in the central structures of the brain)

1090 (FA-394)	Fundamental aspects	HRP in STOMATOLOGICAL DEVELOPMENTS (nociception-antinociception)
Categories of pain - neuropathic (main differences)?		

The differences between such pain and others are :
nociceptive stimulation is intermittent
ineffectiveness of conventional antinociceptive measures
The question of effectiveness is debatable:
nerve blocks
the use of opiates, anxiolytics, anticonvulsants
the use of antidepressants is considered as adjuvant therapy

1091 (FA-395)	Fundamental aspects	HRP in STOMATOLOGICAL DEVELOPMENTS (nociception-antinociception)
Categories of pain - neuropathic (trigeminal neuralgia)?		

Trigeminal neuralgia is one example of neuropathic pain. The distinctive mechanisms of its development are:
demyelination of the fibres of the sensory root at its entrance to the brainstem, associated with atrophy and death of myelin-forming cells - the trigger mechanism
The reasons for this process may be different:

- => inflammation
- => trauma (with subsequent bone changes)
- => extirpation (of teeth, cysts, fistulas)
- => surgeries (jaw and sinus)
- => tumour process
- => prolonged compression by a pulsating vessel

Features of demyelinated fibres:

- => very sensitive (to various agents)
- => have spontaneous activity ("pain paroxysm")
- => create "artificial synapses" and "short circuits" (at the points of contact with each other)

spontaneous "volleys" occur because:

- => permeability of neuronal membranes is disturbed.
- => potassium gradient decreases
- => depolarisation occurs , initiating the repeated discharges

"artificial synapses" on the path from the brainstem to the ganglion determine the return of discharge impulses to the brainstem and its response in the form of repeated increases in discharge; this chain reaction results in the development of very severe pain, which stops only after "exhaustion" of brainstem neurons

1092 (FA-396)	Fundamental aspects	HRP in STOMATOLOGICAL DEVELOPMENTS (nociception-antinociception)
Categories of pain - neuropathic (trigeminal neuritis)?		

The differences in pain in trigeminal neuritis are:

its nature is permanent

such pain is worse when opening the mouth (sharp), eating (hard).

hypoaesthesia in the innervation zone (all types of sensitivity) is manifested, including paresthesias and numbness of the gums, teeth, lips and chin.

in cases of seizure-like course - no facial spasm and convulsions are observed

the neuritis doesn't go away permanently (after a seizure).

In dental practice, the causes of trigeminal neuritis can be:

complex tooth extraction

chronic periodontitis of the mandible

Surgical interventions (mandibular fractures, odontoma, odontogenic cysts)
nerve injury during anaesthesia (conduction)
compression of the inferior alveolar nerve filling material, tooth root fragment, bone breakage, etc.
It can also be caused by narrowing of the bony canals in which the branches of the trigeminal nerve pass:
Acquired (chronic inflammatory processes of teeth, jaw, sinuses)
congenital
Thus, the pathogenetic mechanisms in this affliction may be different:
inflammatory
degenerative
sclerotic
compression
They cause toxic, metabolic and vascular changes in the nerve.

1093 (FA-397)	Fundamental aspects	HRP in STOMATOLOGICAL DEVELOPMENTS (nociception-antinociception)
Categories of pain - neuropathic (phantom pain)?		

Pain in a non-existent (after amputation) limb (so-called "PHANTOM") is explained by the fact that as a result of transection of large nerve trunks, the flow of impulses (through thick fibres) to T-neurons is reduced, which can lead to excitation even from a subthreshold signal.

1094 (FA-398)	Fundamental aspects	HRP in STOMATOLOGICAL DEVELOPMENTS (nociception-antinociception)
Categories of pain - neuropathic (causalgia)?		

If the crossing of a large somatic nerve was incomplete and thick fibres are affected, hyperreactivity of T-neurons occurs because the inhibitory influence of the gelatinous formation is reduced, resulting in "severe" pain. It can be intensified even by minor stimuli (tactile, sound, etc.).

1095 (FA-399)	Fundamental aspects	HRP in STOMATOLOGICAL DEVELOPMENTS (nociception-antinociception)
Categories of pain - neuropathic (glossalgia)?		

To what was said earlier about glossalgia in the previous volumes of this encyclopedia, it should be added that this category of neuropathic pain is polyetiological (observed in pathology of the central nervous system, cardiovascular system, and gastrointestinal tract).

Among dental diseases, it may be noted in:

trigeminal neuritis and neuralgia

traumatic lesion of the inferior alveolar nerve

tongue trauma

other local factors

Clinically observed paresthesia (less often - pain) can be explained by the fact that as a result of excitation of nerve conductors of the tongue and SORP, impulses at the level of reticular formation of the brain are not blocked, but are realised in the form of paresthesias. This usually develops against the background of functional disorders of the CNS.

In this pathology, the phenomena of irritation and trophic disorders may be observed.

Irritation can manifest itself:

paresthesias in one half of the tongue or in the front 2/3 of the tongue, depending on the fibres of the lingual nerve (lingual branch).

Paresthesias on the posterior 1/3 of the tongue and SORP, depending on the lesion of the trigeminal nerve When the tone of the sympathetic nervous system predominates, persistent trophic changes of the tongue and SORP may occur.

It is possible that functional disorders of the antinociceptive system play a role in the pathogenesis of glossalgia.

1096 (FA-400)	Fundamental aspects	HRP in STOMATOLOGICAL DEVELOPMENTS (nociception-antinociception)
Categories of pain - projective (general information)?		

In case of trauma, compression or neuralgia of certain nerves (including facial nerves), the so-called "projection pain" may occur, which is caused by the spread of excitation both in the CNS and to the periphery (in the area of innervation of the sensitive nerve).

1097 (FA-401)	Fundamental aspects	HRP in STOMATOLOGICAL DEVELOPMENTS (nociception-antinociception)
Categories of pain - projective (differential diagnosis)?		

Projective pain should be differentiated from the so-called "reflected" pain, when, as a result of the connection of afferents of the skin and internal organs with the same neurons of the posterior horn of the spinal cord (the beginning of the spinothalamic tract), impulses spread to the corresponding dermatomes.

1098 (FA-402)	Fundamental aspects	HRP in STOMATOLOGICAL DEVELOPMENTS (nociception-antinociception)
Categories of pain - projection pain (tunnel syndrome)?		

The so-called "tunnel" syndrome develops when a peripheral nerve is compressed and selective blockade of impulse conduction along myelinated nerve fibres occurs without affecting unmyelinated primary afferents. The pain response of neurons increases due to the activity of unmyelinated afferents and removal of inhibitory influence - myelinated.

1099 (FA-403)	Fundamental aspects	HRP in STOMATOLOGICAL DEVELOPMENTS (nociception-antinociception)
Categories of pain - terminal (general information)?		

Severe and constant (terminal) pain is seen in:
Oncological diseases (terminal stage)
scleroderma
neuropathies
vascular diseases
AIDS

1100 (FA-404)	Fundamental aspects	HRP in STOMATOLOGICAL DEVELOPMENTS (nociception-antinociception)
Categories of pain - terminal (underlying causes)?		

The main causes of such pain are:

pathogenetic:

- directly in the affected organ (necrosis, infection, ulceration)
- tumour invasion (into bone and periosteum, nerve trunks)
- occlusion of vessels (blood, lymphatic)
- obstruction of an organ (duct)

iatrogenic:

- chemotherapy
- radiotherapy
- postoperative pain
- scar pain

other reasons

- sympathetic reflex dystrophy
- shingles

1101 (FA-405)	Fundamental aspects	HRP in STOMATOLOGICAL DEVELOPMENTS (nociception-antinociception)
Categories of pain - terminal (distinguishing features)?		

The hallmarks of terminal pain are:

■=> alarm
■=> depression
■=> irritation
■=> loss of sleep
■=> fear
■=> the realisation of impending death.

1102 (FA-406)	Fundamental aspects	HRP in STOMATOLOGICAL DEVELOPMENTS (nociception-antinociception)
Categories of pain - terminal (management)?		

The above-mentioned pathogenetic features and distinctive features of terminal pain dictate the need to use not only anti-inflammatory drugs, neuronal blockades, anxiolytics, but also narcotic drugs.
analgesics and antidepressants.

1103 (FA-407)	Fundamental aspects	HRP in STOMATOLOGICAL DEVELOPMENTS (nociception-antinociception)
Categories of pain - chronic?		

In defining pain as "chronic", both the duration of pain syndrome and pain characteristics such as:

■=> predominant relationship with behavioural responses

■=> presence of psychological reactions (neurosis, psychosis, others)

In this regard, narcotic analgesics and anti-inflammatory drugs are contraindicated , and antidepressants are used as adjuvants.

1104 (FA-408)	Fundamental aspects	HRP in STOMATOLOGICAL DEVELOPMENTS (nociception-antinociception)
Categories of pain - psychogenic?		

This type of pain is also possible with dental appointments, but the diagnosis of "psychogenic pain" is only established after a psychiatric counselling, and the psychiatrist determines the patient's treatment plan.

Thus, in order to further define the principles of pain management for different types of pain syndrome, the levels of pain control should be clearly understood.

SEGMENTARY control is characterised by:

it is carried out at the level of the posterior horns of the spinal cord

T cells (transmission) of the gelatinous substance inhibit pain-conducting neurons; this is the so-called "gate principle" when:

o if pain impulsation is conducted predominantly along thick fibres (lemniscus system) gelatinous substance neurons are excited and inhibit T-cell activity (pain is suppressed)

o if pain impulsion is mainly through thin fibres (anterolateral system) gelatinous substance neurons are torqued and their influence on T-cells is inhibited (pain is increased)

The balance of input activation of thick and thin fibres provides the perception of pain intensity

The NADSEGMENTARY control is characterised by the influence on the spinal cord of various subcortical structures of the brain (hypothalamus, suture of the brain stem, etc.), as well as by control from the somatosensory zone of the cortex of the cerebral hemispheres.

LITERATURE

SPECIAL

1. Busygina M.V. Diseases of teeth and mucous membrane of the oral cavity. - Moscow: Medicine, 1967. - 342 c.
2. Grishanin G.G. Stress in stomatology. - Kh.: Caravella, 1998. - 168 c.
3. Dolgikh V.T., Matusov I.E., Chesnokov V.I., Solodnikov N.N., Taran N.I., Korpacheva O.V. Clinical pathophysiology for stomatologist. Edited by Prof. V.T. Dolgikh. - Moscow: Medical Book, N. Novgorod: Izd-vo NGMA, 2000. - 200 c.
4. Limanskiy Y.P. Physiology of pain. - Kiev, 1986. - 93 c.
5. Wounds and wound infection. Manual for doctors / Edited by M.I. Kuzin, V.M. Kostyuchenko. - Moscow: Medicine, 1990. - 592 c.
6. Manual on therapeutic stomatology / Under general ed. by Prof. A.I. Evdokimov. - Moscow: Medicine, 1967. - 572 c.
7. Fedorov Y.A., Volodkina V.V. Treatment of systemic hyperesthesia of dentin in periodontal disease. Methodical letter. - Odessa, 1967. - 14 c.

ADDITIONAL

1. Adaskiewicz V. P. Skin and venereal diseases. - 2nd ed. / V . P. Adaskevich, V. M. Kozin. - Moscow: Medical Literature, 2009. - C. 120-137.
2. Aiziatulov R. F. F. Pustular skin diseases / R. F. Aiziatulov // Journal of Dermatovenerology and Cosmetology named after N. A. Torsuev. N. A. Torsuev. - 2003. - № 1-2. - C. 56-71.
3. Aiziatulov Y. F. Standards of diagnostics and treatment in dermatovenerology / Y. F. Aiziatulov. - Donetsk: Kashtan, 2010. - 560 c.
4. Andrashko Yu. V. Evaluation of the effectiveness of the drug Fuziderm in pustular skin infections and acne / Yu. V. Andrashko, O. M. Galagurich // Ktshchna immunologiya. Alergolopa. 1nfektolopia. - 2007. - № 1. - C. 71-72.
5. Antibacterial therapy: a practical guide / edited by L.S. Strachunsky, Y.B. Belousov, S.N. Kozlov. - Moscow, 2000. - 191 c.
6. Antibacterial drugs in clinical practice: a guide / Edited by S. N. Kozlov, R.S. Kozlov. N. Kozlov, R.S. Kozlov. - Moscow: GEOTAR-Media, 2010. - 232 c.
7. Antibiotic resistance of Streptococcus pyogenes in Russia: results of multicentre prospective study PEGAS-1 / R. S. Kozlov, O. V. Sivaya, K. V. Shpynev, E. D. Agapova [et al] // Clinical Microbiology and

Antimicrobial Chemotherapy. - 2002. - № 4 (2). - C. 154-67.
8. Ataman O. V. Pathological physiology in questions and answers: educational book / O. V. Ataman - 4th edition, stereotype. - Vshnitsa: Nova Kniga, 2010. - 512 c.
9. Buxton P. K. Dermatology / P. K. Buxton. - Moscow: Binom, 2005. - C. 118-122.
10. Belova O. V. V. Immunological function of the skin and neuroimmunocutaneous system / O.V. Belova, V.Y. Arion // Allergology and Immunology. - 2006. - T. 7, № 4. - C. 492-497.
11. Belousova, T. A. Modern principles of external therapy of inflammatory dermatoses / T. A. Belousova // Russian Medical Journal. - 2008. - № 8. - C. 547-551.
12. Belkova Yu. A. Fusidic acid in modern clinical practice (Literature review) / Yu. A. Belkova // Clinical microbiology and antimicrobial chemotherapy. - 2001. - № 4. - C. 324-338.
13. Belyaev G. M. M. Stress, adaptation, psoriasis, planning of scientific research on the problem of this disease / G. M. Belyaev // Dermatolopia ta venerolopia. - 2002. - № 2 (16). - C. 11-14.
14. Byozorov O. P. Detection of gluten enteropathy in psoriasis, allergodermatosis and urogenital chlamyschiasis / O. P. Byozorov // Dermatolopya ta venerolopia. - 2004. - № 2 (24). - C. 29-33.
15. Biochemical parameters in norms and pathology / ed. by O. Y. Sklyarov. - Kyiv: Medicine, 2007. - 318 c.
16. Bolotna L. A. Dryness of shmri: causes and mechanics of development, the possibility of lzhuvalnoe cosmetics / L. A. Bolotna // Dermatolopia ta venerolopia. - 2008. - № 2 (40). - C. 12-17.
17. Bondarenko G. M. Etupatogenesis of Reiter's disease: current status of the problem / G. M. Bondarenko // Dermatolopia ta venereolopia. - 2004. - № 2 (24). - C. 73-80.
18. Burova S. V. Diagnostics of infectious diseases. Part 1. Clinical, clinical-laboratory and instrumental methods / S. V. Burova, M. P. Onukhova, T. Y. Chernobrovkina // International Medical Journal. - 2009. - T. 15, № 1 (57). - C. 127-130.
19. Burova S. V. Diagnostics of infectious diseases. Part 2.
Laboratory special methods / S. V. Burova, M. P. Burova.
Onukhova, T. Y. Chernobrovkina // Clinical, clinical laboratory and instrumental methods International Medical Journal. - 2009. - T. 15, № 2 (58). - C. 113-121.

20. VaryushinaE .A. Studying the mechanisms of the local immunostimulating effect of interleukin-1 in. Enhancement of functional activity of human neutrophil granulocytes in the focus of inflammation under the influence of interleukin-1 in / *E. A.* Varyushina, V. G. Konusova, A. S. Simbirtsev [et al.] // Immunology. - 2000. - № 3. - C. 18-22.
21. Volkova E. N. To the problem of immunopathogenesis of pustular skin diseases / E. N. Volkova Yu. N. To the problem of immunopathogenesis of pustular skin diseases / E. N. Volkova, Y. S. Butov, S. G. Morozov // Vestnik dermatologii i venerologii. - 2004. - № 1. - C. 20-22.
22. Volkoslawska V. M. Status of dermatoses in Ukraine in 20 years after the accident at the Chernobyl accident / V. M. Volkoslawska, O. L. Gugnev, N. O. Chyna // Dermatolopia ta venereolol. - 2009. - № 3 (45). - C. 67-74.
23. Histology (introduction to pathology) / Edited by E.G. Ulumbekov, Yu.A. Chelyshev. - Moscow: GEOTAR MEDICINE, 2005. - 960c.
24. Histopathology and clinical characteristics of dermatoses / G.S. Tseraidis, V.P. Fedotov, A.D. Dyudyun, V.A. Tumansky. - Dnepropetrovsk; Kharkiv; Zaporozhye, 2004. - 536 c.
25. Glukhenky B. T. Pustular skin diseases / B. T. Glukhenky, V. V. Dilektorsky, R. F. Fedorovskaya. - Kiev: Zdorov'ya, 1983. - 136 c.
26. Glukhenkiy B. T. Treatment of patients with dermatological and superficial smooth skin lesions with preparations of a new generation / B. T. Glukhenkiy, A. B. Glukhenka // Ukrainian Journal of Dermatology, Venereology, Cosmetology - 2004. - № 4. - C. 50-52.
27. Goldina O. A. Pyolysin ointment - an effective agent for monotherapy of skin lesions / O. A . Goldina, Yu . V. Gorbachevsky // Poliklinika. - 2009. - №2. - C.84 - 87.
28. Gridasova V. D. Experience of using the drug gatifloxacin (gatibact) in the treatment of pyodermitis / V. D. Gridasova, Z. F. Krivenko // Journal of Dermatovenerology and Cosmetology iM. M. O. Torsueva. - 2006. - № 1-2(12). - C. 222-223.
29. Guchev I. A. Rational antimicrobial chemotherapy of skin and soft tissue infections / I. A. Guchev, S. V. Sidorenko, V. N. Frantsuzov // Antibiotics and Chemotherapy. - 2003. - № 48 (10). - C. 25-31.
30. Dehnich A. V. V. Epidemiology of antibiotic resistance of nosocomial strains of Staphylococcus aureus in Russia: results of a multicentre study / A. V. Dehnich, I. A. Eldelstein, A. D. Narezkina [et al] // Clinical

Microbiology and Antimicrobial Chemotherapy. - 2002. - № 4. - C. 325-336.
31. Dorozhenok I. Yu. Mental disorders provoked by chronic dermatoses: clinical spectrum / I. Yu. Dorozhenok, A. N. Lvov // Vestnik dermatologii i venerologii. - 2009. - № 4. - C. 35-41.
32. Drannik G. N. Clinical immunology and allergology: a manual for students, interns, immunologists, allergists, medical doctors of all specialities / G. N. Drannik. - Kiev: Polygraph Plus LLC, 2010. - 552 c.
33. Dudchenko M. O. Deam factors in the impact of ultrafulet intervals on the width of the tan in prichyaynymi sonyachnyachnogo and piece tanning / M. O. Dudchenko, K. V. Vasilieva, L. Yu Levchenko // Proceedings of the scientific conference "Diseases and age peculiarities of shmri, 1h genetic determshovashstvo". -Conference "Diseases and age specific features of the shmri, 1h genetic determshovashstvo". - Kyiv, 2003. - C. 32-33.
34. Dyudyun A. D. Experience in the treatment of bacterial skin infections with "Floxium" / A. D. Dyudyun. D. Experience in the treatment of bacterial skin infections with the drug "Floxium" / A. D. Dyudyun, N. S. Kolyada, L. A. Pogrebnyak [et al.] // Ukrashskiy jurnal dermatologii, venerologii, kosmetologii. - 2007. - № 3. - C. 61-64.
35. Dyudyun A. D. D. Evaluation of the effectiveness of pyoderma treatment with the use of Fusiderm / A. D. Dyudyun, N. N. Polion, N. D. Getala // Ukrashskiy jurnal dermatologii, venerologii, kosmetologii - 2006. - № 3. - C. 38-40.
36. DyudyunA . D. Fusiderm B in the treatment of patients Allergodermatoses and dermatoses with the presence of bacterial infection / A. D. Dyudyun, N. N. Polion // Ukrashchy Journal of Dermatology, Venereology, Cosmetology - 2006. - № 4. - C. 4245.
37. European Guidelines for the treatment of dermatological diseases: per. from English / ed. by A.D. Katsambasa, T.M. Lotti; per. from English. - Moscow: MEDpress-Inform, 2008. - 736 c.
38. Elisyutina O. G. Role of Staphylococcus aureus in pathogenesis Atopic derm atitis / O. G. Elisyutina, E. S. Fedenko // Russian Allergological Journal. - 2004. - № 1. - C. 1722.
39. Ershov F. I. Interferons and their inducers (from molecules to drugs) / F. I. Ershov, O. I. Kiselev. - Moscow: GOETAR-Media, 2005. - 368 c.
40. Atmospheric pollution and incidence of allergodermatoses in the dry and dry regions of Ukraine / I. I. I. Mavrov, V. M. Volkoslavska, O. L.

Gutnev, O. I. Denisenko // Diseases and age specific features of the population, ix genetic determinability: scientific-practical conference, 2003: theses of the supplements. - Kshv, 2003. - C. 66-69.
41. Zaichenko O. I. Experience of the use of cream "Argosulfan" for treatment of choderms and erosive dermatoses / O. I. Zaichenko. Zaichenko, A. A. Homik, K. F. Vashchenko // Ukrainian Journal of Dermatology, Venereology, Cosmetology. - 2010. - № 1. - C. 37-38.
42. Zinchenko O. B. Influence of antibacterial preparations and means improving peripheral blood circulation on ulcer-necrotic processes in patients with diabetic foot syndrome. Abstract of dissertation ...Candidate of medical sciences, Volgograd. - 2006. - 21c.
43. Immunology / D. Mail, J. Brostoff, D.B. Roth, A. Roit. - Moscow: Logosphere, 2007. - 556 c.
44. Infectious diseases with skin lesions / ed. by Y. V. Lobzin. - SPb: Foliant, 2003. - C. 206-207.
45. Kazmirchuk V. S. Ktshchna immunology and allergy / V. S. Kazmirchuk, L. V. Kovalchuk. - Vshnitsa: Nova Book, 2006. - 526 c.
46. Kalinina N. M. Immunity disorders in relapsing-remitting furunculosis / N. M. Kalinina // Cytokines and inflammation. - 2003. - № 1. - C. 41-44.
47. Kalyuzhnaya L. D. Analysis of the skin microflora of patients with bacterial cellulitis / L. D. Kalyuzhnaya, J. V. Korolova // Dermatovenerology. Cosmetology. Sexopathology. - 2008. - № 1-2 (11). - C. 209-210.
48. Kalyuzhna L. D. Experience in the use of tyrotricin in the treatment of toderms / L. D. Kalyuzhna, M. V. Patel // Dosvshch nauchnogo poshuku young scientists dermatovenerolopov: nauk.-prakt. school, 25 leaffall 2010 p. - Ki! in, 2010. - C. 42.
49. Kalyuzhnaya L. D. Rationale for the use of fusidic acid in the external therapy of atopic dermatitis / L. D. Kalyuzhnaya, E. A. Murzina // Ktshchna immunologiya. Alergolopia. 1nfectolopya. - 2007. - № 4 (9). - C. 1-3.
50. Kamkin A. G. Physiology and molecular biology of cell membranes / A. G. Kamkin. G. Physiology and molecular biology of cell membranes / A. G. Kamkin, I. S. Kiseleva. - Moscow: Academy, 2008. - 592 c.
51. Kamyshnikov V.S. Reference book on clinical and biochemical investigations and laboratory diagnostics / V. S. Kamyshnikov. - 3rd ed. - Moscow: MEDpressinform, 2009. - 896 c.

52. Karsonova M. I. Study of some features of immune status in chronic furunculosis / M. I. Karsonova, J. I. Telnyuk, N. H. Setdikova // Immunopathology, immunology, allergology. - 2002. - № 3. - C. 67-71.
53. Kogan B. G. Rosacea, demodectosis, perioral dermatitis: the most recent aspects of etiology and pathogenesis. New approaches to complex therapy of dermatosis / B.G. Kogan, V.T. Gorgol, V.I. Stepanenko. Stepanenko // Ukrainian Journal of Dermatology, Venereology, Cosmetology. - 2002. - № 4 (7). - C. 50-54.
54. Kozlov V. A. Some aspects of the problem of cytokines / V. A. Kozlov // Cytokines and inflammation. - 2002. - № 1. - C. 5-8.
55. Kozlov P. C. Antibiotic resistance of Streptococcus pyogenes in Russia: results of multicentre prospective study Pegas-I / R. S. Kozlov, O. V. Sivaya, K. V. Shpynev [et al.] // Clin. microbiol. antimicrob. chemother. - 2002. № 4 (2). - C. 154-167.
56. Compendium 2007 - medicinal preparations / ed. by V. N. Kovalenko, A. P. Viktorova. N. Kovalenko, A. P. Viktorov. - Kiev: MORION, 2007. - 2270 c.
57. Korolova Zh. V. Methodology of dermal elasticity examination in patients with unspecified skin defects of the skin, eczema defects, and poor skin / J. V. Korolova, V. V. Vereshchaka // Dermatovenerology. Cosmetology. Sexopathology. - 2008. - № 3-4 (11). - C. 218-221.
58. Korolova Zh. V. Disruptions of blood flow speed in patients with unspecified shdppdrnoT klggkovini infection // J. V. Korolova, V. Vereshchaka // Dermatovenerology . Kosmetologiya. Sexopathology. - 2009. - № 1-2 (12). - C. 31-35.
59. Koshevenko Y. N. Reference book on dermatocosmetology: for doctors and students / Y. N. Koshevenko. - Moscow: Academy of Cosmetology, 2004. - 995c.
60. Kubanova A. A. Methodical materials on diagnosis and treatment of the most common sexually transmitted infections (STIs) and skin diseases. Protocols for the management of patients, drugs / ed. A. A. Kubanova / - Moscow: GEOTAR MEDICINA, 2003 - 87 p.
61. Kubanova A. A. Organisation of dermatological care: achievements and perspectives / A. A. Kubanova, V. A. Martynov, I. H. Lesnaya [et al] // Vestnik dermatologii i venerologii. - 2008. - № 1. - C. 4-22.
62. Kungurov N. V. V. Differentiated external therapy of eczematous manifestations / N. V . Kungurov, M. M. Kohan, Y. V. Keniksfest [et al] //

Medical Technology. - Ekaterinburg, 2007 - 256 p.
63. Kurapov E. P. P. Neurohumoral regulation in patients with systemic inflammatory response syndrome of non-infectious genesis / E. P. Kurapov, I. A. Khripachenko, I. I. Zinkovich // Vestnik hygiene and epidemiology. - 2006. - T. 10, № 1. - 196-204.
64. Kurlovich N. A., Timochko V. R., Kashuba E. A. Blood plasma cytokine levels in staphylococcal infection / N. A. Kurlovich, V. R. Timochko, E. A. Kashuba [et al] // Medical Immunology. - 2006. - № 8 (2-3). - C. 276-277.
65. Kurchenko A. I. The role of Langerhans cells in the yunshi system of shmri / A. I. Kurchenko. Kurchenko // Ukrainian Journal of Dermatology, Venereology, Cosmetology. - 2001. - № 2-3. - C. 6-9.
66. Kutasevich Ya. F. Place of external preparations containing fusidic acid in the treatment of infectious inflammatory diseases of the skin and soft tissues / J. F. Kutasevich, A. N. Ogurtsova // Dermatolopia ta venerolopia. - 2007. - № 1. - C. 5358.
67. Kutasevich Ya. F. New possibilities of treatment of bacterial skin infections / J. F. Kutasevich, A. N. Ogurtsova // Novosti meditsiny i pharmacii. - 2008. - № 7. - C. 3-4.
68. Lebedev K. A. Immune insufficiency (detection and treatment) / K. A. Lebedev, I. D. Ponyakina. - Moscow: Izd-vo NGMA, 2003. - 442 c.
69. Lomonosov K. M. Oxidative stress and antioxidant therapy in various skin diseases / K. M. Lomonosov // Russian journal of skin and venereal diseases. - 2009. - № 2. - C. 27-31.
70. Mavrov G. I. Pathogenetic therapy of patients with resistant herpes, chlamydia and syphilis by regulating cytokshovogo profile: Methodical recommendations / G. I. Mavrov, G. M. Bondarenko, G. P. Chshov [and in. Mavrov, G. M. Bondarenko, G. P. Chshov [and in.]. - Kiev, 2005. - 23 c.
71. Mavrov I. I. Fundamentals of diagnosis and treatment in dermatology and venereology: a guide for doctors, interns, students / I. I. Mavrov, L. A. Bolotnaya, I. M. Serbina. - Kharkov: Fakt, 2007. - 792 c.
72. Mavrov I. I. Efficacy and tolerability of ceftriaxone in combination with sulbactam in the treatment of complicated statin infection caused by pathogenic bacteria / I. I.I. Mavrov, L. V. Bashchenko // Dermatolopaia and Venereolopaia. I.I. Mavrov, L.V. Bashchenko // Dermatology and Venereology. - 2009. - № 1 (43). - C. 42-46.
73. Masyukova S. A. Bacterial skin infections and their significance in the

clinical practice of a dermatologist / S. A. Masyukova, V. V. Gladko, M. V. Ustinov [et al] // Consilium medicum. - 2004. - № 6 (3). - C. 180-185.
74. Masyukova SA Fusidic acid in the treatment of pyelodermitis and allergodermatosis complicated by bacterial infection / S. A. Masyukova, V. V. Gladko, G. N. Tarasenko et al. // Vestnik dermatologii i venerologii. - 2007. - № 6. - C. 54-57.
75. Medical microbiology: textbook / ed. by V. I. Pokrovsky. I. Pokrovsky. - Moscow: GEOTAR-Media, 2008. - 768 c.
76. MedunitsynN . V. Fundamentals of immunoprophylaxis and Immunotherapy of infectious diseases: textbook / N. V. Medunitsyn, V. I. Pokrovsky. - Moscow: GE OTAR-Media, 2005. - 512 c.
77. Metals in osteoarthritis / ed. by O. V. Sinyachenko. - Donetsk: Nord-Press, 2008. - 404 c.
78. Moibenko M. Mupirocin: an antibiotic with a unique structure for topical application / M. Moibenko // Ukrashskiy Zhurnal Dermatologii, Venerologii, Kosmetolopi - 2009. - № 2. - C. 3942.
79. Nerush O. P. Pyococcal infection - a complicating course of neurodermatitis / O. P. Nerush // Dermatovenerology. Cosmetology. Sexopathology. - 2004. - № 1-2 (7). - C. 212213.
80. Novikov A. I. Skin diseases of infectious and parasitic origin. Manual for doctors / ed. A. I. Novikov, E. A. Loginova. - Moscow: Medical Book, 2001. - 450 c.
81. Novoselov V. S. Pyoderma / V. S. Novoselov, L. R. Plieva // Russian Medical Journal. - 2004. - T. 12, №5. - C. 327335.
82. Ogurtsova AN Differentiated approach to the treatment of acne / AN Ogurtsova // Actual issues of dermatovenerology and cosmetology: scientific and practical conference abstract - Odessa, 2003. - C. 83-84.
83. Oleinik I. A. Hepatotropic effect of thiotriazolin in the treatment of chronic dermatoses / I. A. Oleinik, L. V.
Ivashchenko, V. V. Gun'kova // Journal of Dermatovenerology and Cosmetology named after N. A. Torsuev. N. A. Torsuev. - 2004. - № 1-2 (8). - C. 133134.
84. Olshnik I. O. Peculiarities of gastko tissue remodelling in arthropathic psorchia and methods of its correction / I. O. Olshnik // Dermatololya ta venereololya. O. Olshnik // Dermatolol ta venerololol. - 2009. - № 1 (43). - C. 20-24.
85. Fundamentals of clinical immunology / E. Chepel, M. Haney, S. Misbah, N. Snovden; per. from Engl. 5th ed. - Moscow: GEOTAR-Media,

2008. - 416 c.
86. Assessment of staphylococcal and non-lipophilic yeast microflora of the skin in patients with skin pathology by contact method of seeding / V. G. Arzumanyan, E. V. Zaitseva, T. N. Kabaeva, R. V. Temper // Vestnik dermatologii i venerologii. - 2004. - № 6. - C. 3.
87. Paltsev M. A., Kvetnoy I. M. Manual on neuroimmunoendocrinology / M. A. Paltsev, I. M. Kvetnoy. - Moscow: Medicine, 2006. - 384 c.
88. Patent for corisnu model 47304 Ukrania, MPK[51] A61K31/7105. Spoab lshuvannya chromechnyh recidivuyuchikh todermsh / V.A. Bocharov, V.V. Gun'kova, A.Y. Askevich, V.V. Bocharova [and in.], applicant and patent holder Zaporizkiy State Medical University. - Published 25.01.2010, Bulletin No. 2.
89. Petri A. Clear medical statistics / A. Petri, K. Sabin; translated from English, ed. by V. P. Leonov. P. Leonov. - 2nd ed., revision and addendum - Moscow: GEOTAR-Media, 2010. - 168 c.
90. Pogrebnyak L. A. Experience in the use of Fromilide in the treatment of pyoderma in children / L. A. Pogrebnyak. A. Pogrebnyak, E.K. Kostromtsova, Yu.
Belozerskaya //. Dermatovenerology. Cosmetology. Sexopathology. - 2004. - № 1-2 (7). - C. 220-221.
91. Protsenko T. V. Influence of sex hormones on physiological processes in the dermis / T. V. Protsenko, I. N. Bondarenko // Dermatovenerology. Cosmetology. Sexopathology. - 2001. - № 1 (4). - C. 133-137.
92. Psyuk S.K. Effectiveness of antifungin in the treatment of pyoderma / S.K. Psyuk, S.A. Bondar, I.N. Lyashenko [et al] // Dermatovenerology. Cosmetology. Sexopathology. - 2008. - № 1-2 (11). - C. 292-293.
93. Pyatikop I. A. Experience of using Ketozoral-Darnica cream in external therapy of patients with microsporia / I. A. Pyatikop, I. V. Kadygrob, T. V. Zimina [et al] // Dermatovenerology. Cosmetology. Sexopathology. - 2004. - № 1-2 (7). - C. 203-204.
94. Radionov V. G. Prospects for the use of Orungal for the prevention of biological complications of antibiotic therapy / V. G. Radionov, I. P. Belousova // Dermatovenerology. Cosmetology. Sexopathology. - 2001. - № 2-3 (4). - C. 33-35.
95. Рахманов P. S. On the role of natural resistance of the organism in the prevention of pustular skin diseases among persons of the organised military collective / R. S. Rakhmanov, M. A. Medzhidova // Zdravookhranenie Rossiyskoy Federatsii. - 2007. - № 4. - C. 51-52.

96. Rational antimicrobial pharmacotherapy / ed. by V. P. Yakovlev, S. V. Yakovlev. P. Yakovlev, S. V. Yakovlev. - Moscow: Littera, 2003. - C. 102-110, 369-378.
97. Rational pharmacotherapy of skin diseases and sexually transmitted infections: a handbook for practitioners /
A. A. Kubanova, V. I. Kisina, L. A. Blatun, A. M. Vavilov [et al.]; ed. by A. A. Kubanova, V. I. Kisina. - Moscow: Litterra, 2005. - 882 c.
98. Rozum I. A. Derinat in the treatment of patients with nasal furunculosis / I. A. Rozum // Vestnik otorhinolaryngologii. - 2002. - № 5. - C. 12-15.
99. The role of immune st atus in the pathogenesis of acne disease / A. N. Ogurtsova, I. A. Mashtakova, L. S. Tatskaya, E. N. Soloshenko // Dermatovenerology. Cosmetology. Sexopathology. - 2004. - № 1-2 (7). - C. 215.
100. Samgin MA New opportunities in the treatment of atopic dermatitis and pyoderma / MA Samgin, SA Monakhov //Doctor Ru. - 2006. - № 1. - C. 40-41.
101. Svirid S.G. Immune status of women suffering from urogenital infections / S.G. Svirid, S.E. Mokretsov // Dermatovenerology. Cosmetology. Sexopathology. - 2002. - № 1-2 (5). - C. 86-88.
102. Svyatenko T.V. Dermatoses complicated by secondary infection: emphasis on external therapy / T.V. Svyatenko, O.S. Dudnik, A .A. Frankenberg // Dermatovenerology.
Cosmetology. Sexopathology. - 2009. - № 1-2 (12). - C. 268272.
103. Svyatenko T. V. Modern opportunities and near future prospects in the treatment of bacterial skin infections / T. V. Svyatenko, M. A. Nikolaychuk, A. A. Frankenberg // Ukrainian Journal of Dermatology, Venereology, Cosmetology. - 2010. - № 2. - C. 23-28.
104. Sepiashvili R.I. Fundamentals of physiology of the immune system / R.I. Sepiashvili. - Moscow: Medicine, 2003. - 239 c.
105. Sergeev A. Yu. Immunoderm atology: immunological bases of pathogenesis of the main inflammatory dermatoses of man / A. Yu. Sergeev, A. V. Karaulov, Y. V. Sergeev // Immunology, Allergology, Infectology. - 2003. - № 3. - C. 10-23.
106. Sergeev Yu. V. New approaches to local therapy of pyoderma and complicated dermatoses / Yu. V. Sergeev, V. N. Larionova, P. V. Kamennenykh [et al.] // Clinical Dermatology and Venereology. - Moscow. - 2008. - № 6. - C. 55-58.

107. Simbirtsev A. C. Cytokines - a new system of regulation of defence reactions of the organism / A. S. Simbirtsev // Cytokines and inflammation. - 2002. - №1 (1). - C. 9-16.
108. Simbirtsev A. C. Cytokines: classification and biological functions / A. S. Simbirtsev // Cytokines and inflammation. - 2004. - № 3 (2). - C. 16-21.
109. Skripkin Yu. K. Skin and venereal diseases / Y.K. Skripkin, A.A. Kubanova, V.G. Akimov. - Moscow: GEOTAR-Media, 2009. - C. 103-127.
110. Skripkin Yu. K. Skin and venereal diseases: a pupil for doctors and students of medical universities / Y. K. Skripkin. - Moscow: Triada-farm, 2001. - 688 c.
111. Skripkin Yu. K. Experience of using Oxycort and Polcortolon TS aerosols in the treatment of allergic dermatoses, weakened by pyoderma / Y. K. Skripkin, I. V. Khamaganova // Bulletin of Dermatology and Venereology. - 2004. - № 1. - C. 42-43.
112. Soloshenko E. M. Diagnosis and basic principles of rational therapy of secondary immunodeficiencies at Dermatovenerological practices: methodological recommendations / E. M. Soloshenko, M. M. Popov. - Krzw, 2003. - 16 c.
113. Sorokina E. V. V. Features of immunological status in patients with pyoderma: Review / E. V. Sorokina, E. A. Kurbatova, S. A. Masyukova // Bulletin of Dermatology and Venereology. - 2005. - № 5. - C. 4-10.
114. Stepanenko V. I. Urogenggalsh shfektsl: trichomoshaz, candidiasis, geshalnyi herpes / V. I. Stepanenko, T. S. Konovalova. - Krzw: K1M Publishing House, 2008. - 288 c.
115. StrachunskyL . S. Comparative activity Antibacterial preparations included in dosage forms for topical use against Staphylococcus aureus: results of the Russian multicentre study PEGAS-1 / L. S. Strachunsky, A. V. Dehnich, Y. A. Belkova // Clinical Microbiology and Antimicrobial Chemotherapy. - 2002. T. 4, № 2. - C. 157-163.
116. Sudakov K. V. Normal physiology / K. V. Sudakov. - Moscow: LLC "Medical Information Agency", 2006. - 920 c.
117. File T. Diagnosis and antimicrobial therapy of skin and soft tissue infections (lecture) / T. File // Clinical Microbiology and Antimicrobial Chemotherapy. - USA, Ohio. - № 2, T. 5. - 2003.
118. Fedotov V. P. Experience in the use of cream "Lom eksin" in

external therapy of bacterial and fungal skin diseases / V. P. Fedotov, V. V. Gorbuntsov, O. P. Benyukh // Dermatovenerology. Cosmetology. Sexopathology. - 2009. - № 1-2 (12). - C. 264-267.
119. Khaldin A. A. A. Rational antibacterial therapy in the practice of dermatovenerologist / A. A. Khaldin // Russian Medical Journal. - 2005. - T. 13, № 5. - C.273-277.
120. Shevela A. G. Experience of using antiseptic paste "Antisept" in streptoderma / A. G. Shavela, S. Z. Vitenchuk, O. V. Fenenko // Dermatovenerology. Cosmetology.
Sexopathology. - 2005. - № 3-4(8). - C. 215.
121. Chancriform pyoderma (case description) / I.V. Kuleshov, V.N. Lin, G.L. Krulenko, N.N. Tsabak // Dermatovenerology. Cosmetology. Sexopathology. - 2004. - № 1-2 (7). - C. 151-152.
122. Shlyapnikov S. A. Use of macrolides in surgical infections of skin and soft tissues / S . A. Shlyapnikov, V. V. Fedorova // Russian Medical Journal. - 2004. - T. 12. - № 4. - C. 204-207.
123. Yushchishin N. I. Bacterial immunostimulants in the treatment of chronic pyoderma in children / N. I. Yushchishin // Dermatovenerology. Cosmetology. Sexopathology. - 2009. - № 1-2 (12). - C. 345-347.
124. Yakovlev S. V. Azithromycin: basic properties,
Optimisation of modes of application based on pharmacokinetic and pharmacodynamic parameters / S. V. Yakovlev, S. A. Ukhtin // Antibiotics and Chemotherapy. - 2003, T. 48, № 2. - C. 22-27.
125. Afset J. E. Susceptibility of skin and soft-tissue isolates of Staphylococcus aureus and Streptococcus pyogenes to topical antibiotics: indications of clonal spread of fusidic acid-resistant Staphylococcus aureus / J. E. E. Afset, J. A. Maeland // Scand. J. Infect. Dis. - 2003. - V. 35, № 2. - P. 84-89.
126. Birnkrant M. J. Pyoderma gangrenosum, acne conglobata, and IgA gammopathy / M. J. Birnkrant, A. J. Papadopoulos, R. A. Schwartz [et al] // Int. J. Birnkrant, A. J. Papadopoulos, R. A. Schwartz [et al.] // Int. J. Dermatol. - 2003. - V. 42, № 3. - P. 213- 216.
127. Bisno A. L. Streptococcus pyogenes / A. L. Bisno, D. L. Stevens // In: Mandell G. L., Bennett J. E., Dolin R. editors. Mandell, Douglas, and Bennett's principles and practice of infectious diseases. 6th ed. Philadelphia: Churchill Livingston. - 2005. - P. 2362-2379.
128. Chavakis T. Staphylococcus aureus extracellular adherence protein serves as anti-inflammatory factor by inhibiting the recruitment of host

leukocytes / T. Chavakis, M. Hussain, S. M. Kanse [et al.] // Nat. Med. - 2002. V. 8. - P. 687-93.
129. Eady A. A. Staphylococcal resistance revisited: community-acquired methicillin resistant Staphylococcus aureus - an emerging problem for the management of skin and soft tissue infections / A. A. A. Eady, J. H. Cove // Curr. Opin. Infect. Dis. - 2003. - V. 16. - P. 10324. Elston D. M. Epidemiology and prevention of skin and soft tissue infections cutis / D. M. Elston. - 2004. - 73 (Suppl 5). P. 3-7.
130. Effect of farnesol on Staphylococcus aureus biofilm formation and antimicrobial susceptibility / M. A. Jabra-Rizk, T. F. Meiller, C. E. James, M. E. Shirtlift // Antimicrob. Agents Chemother. - 2006. - V. 50, № 4. - P. 1463-1469.
131. Eguchi K. Apoptosis in autoimmune diseases / K. Eguchi // Inter. Eguchi // Inter. Med. - 2001. - V. 40, № 4. - P. 275-284.
132. Elston D. M. Epidemiology and prevention of skin and soft tissue infections / D. M. M. Elston // Cutis. - 2004. - V. 73 (Suppl 5). - P. 3-7.
133. Eron L. J. Managing skin and soft tissue infection: expert panel recommendations key decision points / L. J. Eron. J. Eron., B. A. Lipsky, D. E. Low [et al.] // J. Antimicrob. Chemother. - 2003. - V. 52 (Suppl. Sl). - P. 13-117.
134. Faergemann J. Seborrhoeic dermatitis and Pityrosporum (Malassezia) folliculitis: characterisation of inflammatory cells and mediators in the skin by immunohistochemistry / J. Faergemann J. Faergemann, I. M. Bergbrant, M. Dohse [et al.] // Br. J. Dermatol. - 2001. - V. 144, № 3. - P. 549-556.
135. Fey P. D. Comparative molecular analysis of community- or hospital-acquired methicillin-resistant Staphylococcus aureus / P. D. Fey, B. Said-Salim, M. E. Rupp [et al.] // Antimicrob. Agents. Chemother. - 2003. - V. 47. - P. 96-203.
136. Foster T. J. Surface protein adhesins of Staphylococcus aureus / T. J. Foster, M. Hook // Trends Microbiol. - 1998. - V. 6 (484) - P. 484-488.
137. Frazee B. W. High prevalence of methicillin-resistant Staphylococcus aureus in emergency department skin and soft tissue infections / B. W. Frazee, J. Lynn, E. D. Charlebois [et al.] // Ann. Emerg. Med. - 2005. - V. 45. - P. 311-20.
138. Furunculosis and Ig G subclass deficiency / E. Mahe, N. Girzin, V. Descamps, B. Crickx // Dermatology. - 2004. - V. 208, № 1. - P. 84-85.
139. Gilbert D. N. The Sanford Guide to Antimicrobial Therapy / D. N.

N. Gilbert, R. C. Moellering Jr., G. M. Eliopoulos [et al.]. - 35th ed. New York: Atimicrobial Therapy, 2005.
140. Gosbell I. B. Community-acquired, non-multiresistant oxacillinresistant Staphylococcus aureus (NORSA) in south western Sydney / I. B. Gosbell, J. L. Mercer, S. A. Neville R. [et al.] // Pathology. - 2001. - V. 33, № 2. - P. 206-210.
141. Gosbell I. B. Methicillin-resistant Staphylococcus aureus impact on dermatology practice / I. B. B. Gosbell // Am. J. Clin. Dermatol. - 2004. V. 5, № 239. - P. 59.
142. Gotz F. Staphylococcus and biofilms / F. Gotz // Mol. Microbiol. - 2002. - V. 43. - P. 1367-78.
143. Grundmeier M. Truncation of fibronectin-binding proteins in Staphylococcus aureus strain Newman leads to deficient adherence and host cell invasion due to loss of the cell wall anchor function / M. Grundmeier. Grundmeier, M. Hussain, P. Becker // Infect. Immun. - 2004. - V. 120. - P. 7155-7163.
144. Guerin F. Outbreak of methicillin-resistant Staphylococcus aureus with reduced susceptibility to glycopeptides in a Parisian hospital / F. Guerin. Guerin, A. Buu-Hoi, J.-L. Mainardi [et al.] // J. Clin. Clin. Microbiol. - 2000. - V. 38 - P. 2985-8.
145. Hou D. X. Involvement of reactive oxygen species-independent mitochondrial pathway in gossypol-induced apoptosis / D. X. Hou, T. Uto, X. Tong [et al.] // Arch. Biochem. Biophys. - 2004. - V. 428, № 2. - P. 179-187.
146. Inha B. Heterologously expressed staphylococcus aureus fibronectin-binding proteins are sufficient for invasion of host cells / B. Inha. Inha, P. Francois // Infect. Immun. - 2000. - V. 68. - P. 68716878.
147. Janeway C. A. Innate immune recognition / C. A. Janeway, R. Madzhitov // Ann. Rev. Immunol. - 2002. - V. 20. - P. 197-216.
148. Jones M. E. Epidemiology and antibiotic susceptibility of bacteria causing skin and soft tissue infections in the United States and Europe: a guide to appropriate antimicrobial treatment / M. E. E. Jones, J. A. Karlowskv, D. C. Draghi [et al.] // Int. J. Antimicrob. Agent. - 2003. - V. 22. - P. 406-419.
149. Jones P. G. Mupirocin resistance in clinical isolates of Staphylococcus aureus / P. G. Jones, T. Sura, M. Harris [et al.] // Infect. Control. Hosp. Epidemiol. - 2003. - V. 24 (4). - P. 300-30l.
150. Kallen A. Increase in community-acquired methicillin-resistant

Staphylococcus aureus at a naval medical centre / A. Kallen. Kallen, O. Driscoll, S. Thornton [et al.] // Infect. Control. Hosp. Epidemiol. - 2000. - V. 21. - P. 223-6.
151. Kaviratne M. IL-13 activates mechanism of tissue fibrosis that is completely TGF-beta independent / M. Kaviratne, M. Hesse, M. Leusink [et al.] // J. Immunol. Immunol. - 2004. - V. 173. - P. 4020-4029.
152. Kensuke M. Innate immune sensing of pathogens and danger signals by cell surface Toll-like receptors / Kensuke M. // Sem. Immunol. - 2007. - V. 19. - P. 3-10.
153. Kepler T. Spatiotemporal programming of a simple inflammatory process / T. Kepler, C. Chan // Immunol. Rev. - 2007. - V. 216, № 1. - P. 153-163.
154. Khan I. A. Interleukin-12 enhances murine survival against acute toxoplasmosis / I. A. Khan, T. Matsuura, L. H. Kasper // J. Virol. Virol. 2003. - V 77, № 13. - P. 7444-7451.
155. Kim J. Activation of toll-like receptor in acne triggers inflammatory cytokine responses / J. Kim. Kim, M. T. Ochoa, S. R. Krutzik [et al.] // J. Immunol. Immunol. - 2002. - V. 16, № 3. - P. 1535-1541.
156. Komisarenko S. Lymphocyte activation - from the surface to the nucleus / S. Komisarenko // Ukrainian Biochemical Journal. - 2005. - T. 77, № 2. - C. 8.
157. Kovalchuk L. V. Herpes simplex virus: treatment with antimicrobial peptides / Kovalchuk L.V., Gankovskaja L.V., Gankovskaja O.A.. [et al.] // Adv. Exp. Med. Biol. - 2007. - V. 601. - P. 369-376.
158. Kreikemeyer B. Streptococcus pyogenes fibronectin-binding protein F2: expression profile, binding characteristics, and impact on eukaryotic cell interactions / B. Kreikemeyer, S. Oehmcke, M. Nakata [et al. Kreikemeyer, S. Oehmcke, M. Nakata [et al.] // J. Biol. Biol. Chem. - 2004. - V. 279. - P. 15850-15859.
159. Kupper T. S. Immune surveillance in the skin: mechanisms and clinical consequences / T. S. Kupper, R. C. Fuhlbrigge // Nat. Rev. Immunol. - 2004. - V. 7. - P. 211-222.
160. Laube S. Bacterial skin infections in the elderly: diagnosis and treatment / S. Laube, A. M. Farrel // Drugs Aging. - 2002. - V. 19, № 5. - P. 331-342.
161. Life span of skin homing T cells in atopic dermatitis: survival in skin, activation induced apoptosis in peripheral blood / M. Akdis. Akdis, A. Trautmann, K. Blaser, C.A. Akdis // J. Allergy Clin. Allergy Clin.

Immunol. - 2000. - V. 105. - P. 167.
162. Managing skin and soft tissue infection: expert panel recommendations key decision points / L. J. Eron, B. A. Lipsky, D. E. Low [et al.] // J. Antimicrob. Chemother. - 2003. V. 52 (Suppl. S1). - P. 13-117.
163. Medzhitov R. Innate immunity / R. Medzhitov, C. Janeway // N. Engl. Engl. J. Med. - 2000. - V. 343, № 5. - P. 338-344.
164. Meyers B. R. Antimicrobial Therapy Guide / B. R. Meyers. editor. 16th ed. - Newtown: Antimicrobial Prescribing, 2004.
165. Misery L. How the skin reacts to environmental factors / L. Misery // JEADV. - 2007. - V. 21, № 2. - P. 5-7.
166. Moreillon P. Staphylococcus aureus (Including Staphylococcal Toxic Shock) / P. Moreillon, Y.-A. Que, M. P. Glauser // In: Mandell G. L., Bennett J. E., Dolin R., ed. Mandell, Douglas, and Bennett's principles and practice of infectious diseases. 6th ed. Philadelphia: Churchill Livingston. - 2005. - P. 2321-2351.
167. Mupirocin resistance in clinical isolates of Staphylococcus aureus / P. G. Jones, T. Sura, M. Harris, A. Strother // Infect. Control. Hosp. Epidemiol. - 2003. - № 24. - P. 300-301.
168. Murakawa G. J. Common pathogens and differential diagnosis of skin and soft tissue infections / G. J. Murakawa // Cutis. J. Murakawa // Cutis. - 2004. - V. 73 (Suppl 5). - P. 7-10.
169. Nishijima S. Antimicrobial resistance of Staphylococcus aureus isolated from skin infections / S. Nishijima, I. Kurokawa // Int. J. Antimicrob. Agents. - 2002. - V. 19 (3) - P. 241-3.
170. Niyonsaba F. Human defensins and cathelicidins in the skin: beyond direct antimicrobial properties / F. Niyonsaba, I. Nagaoka, H. Ogawa // Crit. Niyonsaba, I. Nagaoka, H. Ogawa // Crit. Rev Immunol. - 2006. - № 26 (6). - P. 545-547.
171. Nizet V. Innate antimicrobial peptide protects the skin from invasive bacterial infection / V. Nizet, T. Ohtake, X. Lauth [et al.] // Nature. - 2001. - V. 414. - P. 454-457.
172. Okuma K. Dissemination of new methicillin-resistant Staphylococcus aureus clones in the community / K. Okuma K. Iwakawa K, J. D. Turnidge [et al. Okuma, K. Iwakawa K, J. D. Turnidge [et al.] // J. Clin. Clin. Microbiol. - 2002. - V. 40. - P. 4289-94.
173. O'Neill A. J. Mutation frequencies for resistance to fusidic acid and rifampicin in Staphylococcus aureus / A. J. J. O'Neill, J. H. Cove, I. J.

Chopra // Antimicrob. Chemother. - 2001. - V. 47. -P. 647-650.
174. Outbreaks of community-associated methicillin-resistant Staphylococcus aureus skin infections. - Los Angeles County, California. 2002-2003. - V. 52, № 5. - P. 88.
175. Perez-Fontan M. Mupirocin resistance after long term use for Staphylococcus aureus colonisation in patients undergoing chronic peritoneal dialysis / M. Perez-Fontan. Perez-Fontan, M. Rosales, A. Rodriguez-Carmona [et al.] // Am. J. Kidney Dis. - 2002. - V. 39, № 2. - P. 337-341.
176. Reitano S. Topical noncorticosteroid immunomodulation in the treatment of atopic dermatitis / S. Reitano, A. Remitz, Kyllonen // Am. Reitano, A. Remitz, Kyllonen // Am. J. Clin. Dermatol. - 2002. - V. 3. - P. 381-388.
177. Rennie R. P. SENTRY Programme Study Group (North America). Occurrence and antimicrobial susceptibility patterns of pathogens isolated from skin and soft tissue infections: report from the SENTRY Antimicrobial Surveillance Programme (United States and Canada, 2000) / R. P. Rennie, R. N. Jones, A. H. Mutnick // Diagnosis. P. Rennie, R. N. Jones, A. H. Mutnick // Diagn. Microbiol. Infect. Dis. - 2003. - V. 45. - P. 287-293.
178. Rist T. A comparison of the efficacy and safety of mupirocin cream and cephalexin in the treatment of secondarily infected eczema / T. Rist, L. C. Parish, L. C., L. R. Capin [et al.] // Clin. Exp. Dermatol. - 2002. - V. 27, № 1. - P. 14-20.
179. Rohani M. Y. Susceptibility pattern of Staphylococcus aureus isolated in Malaysian hospitals / M. Y. Y. Rohani, A. Raudzah, M. G. Lau [et al.] // Int. J. Antimicrob. Agents. - 2000. -V. 13. - V. 209213.
180. Rothoeft T. Antigen dose, type of antigen-presenting cell end time of differentiation contribute to the T helper 1 / T helper 2 polarisation of nave T cells / T. Rothoeft, F. Gonschorec, H. Bartz [et al.] // Immunology. - 2003. - V. 110. - P. 430-439.
181. Sader H. S. SENTRY Participants Group (Latin America). Skin and soft tissue infections in Latin American medical centres: four-year assessment of the pathogen frequency and antimicrobial susceptibility patterns // H. S. Sader, R. N. Jones, J. B. Silva // Diagn. Microbiol. Infect. Dis. - 2002. - V. 44 (3). - P. 281-8.
182. Saigado C. D. Community-acquired methicillin-resistant Staphylococcus aureus: A meta-analysis of prevalence and risk factors / C.

D. D. Saigado, B. M. Farr, D. P. Calfee // Clin. Infect. Dis. - 2003. - V. 36. - P. 131-9.
183. Schauber J. Antimicrobial peptides and the skin immune defence system / J. Schauber. Schauber, R. L. Gallo // J. Allergy Clin. Allergy Clin. Immunol. - 2008. - № 122 (2). - P. 261-266.
184. Serhan C. N. Resolution phase of inflammation: nevel endogenous anti-inflammatory and proresolving lipid mediators and pathways / C. N. Serhan // Ann. Rev. Immunol. - 2007. - V. 25. - P. 101-137.
185. Simon R. Is a Staphylococcus aureus is a broad spectrum, iron-regulated adhesion / R. Simon, D. Michael // Mol. Microbiol. - 2004. - V. 51. - P. 1509-1519.
186. Skov L. Bacterial superan-tigens and inflammatory skin diseases / L. Skov, O. Baadsgaard // Clin. Exp. Dermatol. - 2000. - V. 25. - P. 57-61.
187. Stevens D. L. Practice guidelines for the diagnosis and management of skin and soft-tissue infections / D. L. Stevens, A. L.
Bisno, H. F. Chambers [et al.] // Clin. Infect. Dis. - 2005. - V. 41. - P. 1373-406.
188. Stockfleth E. Illuminating the mode of action of Toll-like receptor-7 and -8 agonist in dermatology // Arzneim-Forsch. - 2007. - V. 51, № 1. - P. 73.
189. Stratchounski L. S. Antimicrobial resistence of nosocomical strains of Staphylococcus aureus in Russia: results of prospective study / L. S. Stratchounski. S. Stratchounski, A. V. Dekhnich , V. A. Kretchlkov [et al.] // J. Chem. Chemother. - 2005. - V. 17 (1). - P. 54-60.
190. Stulberg D. L. Common bacterial skin infections / D. L. Stulberg, M. A. Penrod, R. A. Blatny // Am. Fam. Physician. - 2002. - V. 66, № 1. - P. 119-124.
191. Swartz M. N. Cellulitis and subcutaneous tissue infection / M. N. Swartz, M. S. Pasternack // In: Mandell G. L., Bennett J. E., Dolin R., ed. Mandell, Douglas, and Bennett's principles and practice of infectious diseases. 6th ed. Philadelphia: Churchill Livingston. - 2005. - P. 1172-1193.
192. Taylor P. R. Macrophage receptors and immunorecognition / P. R. Taylor, L. Martinez-Pomares, M. Stacey [et al.] // Ann. Rev. Immunol. - 2005. - V. 23. - P. 901-944.
193. Tristan A. Use of multiplex PCR to identify Staphylococcus aureus adhesions' involved in human hematogenous infections / A. Tristan, L. Ying, M. Bes // J. Clin. Clin. Microbiol. - 2003. - V. 41. - P. 4465-4467.

194. Tulic M. K. TLR4 polymorphism's mediate impaired response to respiratory syncytial virus and lipopolysaccharide / M. K. Tulic, R. J. Hurrelbrink, C. M. Prele [et al.] // J. Immunol. Immunol. - 2007. - V. 179. - P. 132-140.

195. Wacim A. N. Influence of thyroxine on human granulose cell in vitro / A. N. Wacim, S. L. Polizotto, D. R. Burholt // J. Assist Reprod Genet. - 2001. - V. 12. - P. 274-277.

196. Walton S. The acne in adults / S. Walton, W. J. Cunliffe, A. S. Early // Brit. J. Dermatol. - 1995. - V. 133. - P. 249-253.

197. Webster G. F. Acne vulgaris: State of the science / G. F. F. Webster // Arch. of Dermatol. - 2001. - № 135. - P. 1101-1109.

198. Weems J. J. Nasal Carriage of Staphylococcus aureus as a risk factor for skin and soft tissue infections / J. J. Weems. J. Weems, L. B. Beck // Curr. Infect. Dis. Rep. - 2002. - V. 4. - P. 420-5.

199. Wehner J. Staphylococcus aureus enterotoxins induce histamine and leukotreene release in patients with atopic eczema / J. Wehner, K. Neuber // Br. J. Dermatol. - 2001. - V. 2. - P. 302-305.

200. Wilson D.H.. Health status of hormone replacement therapy users and non-users as determined by the quality-of-life dimension / D. H. Wilson, A. W. Taylor, A. H. Lennan // J. of the International Menopause Society. H. Wilson, A. W. Taylor, A. H. Lennan // J. of the International Menopause Society. - New York-London, 2002. -V. l, No. l. - P. 5055.

201. Yacoubian S. New endogenous anti-inflammatory and proresolving lipid mediators: implication for rheumatic disease / S. Yacoubian, C. N. Serhan // Nat. Clin. Pract. Rheumatic. - 2007. - V. 3. - P. 570-579.

202. Yamasaki O. Clinical manifestation of staphylococcal scalded-skin syndrome depend on serotypes of exfoliative toxins / O. Yamasaki, T. Yamaguchi, M. Sugai [et al. Yamasaki, T. Yamaguchi, M. Sugai [et al.] // J. Clin. Clin. Microbiol. - 2005. - V. 43. - P. 1890-1893.

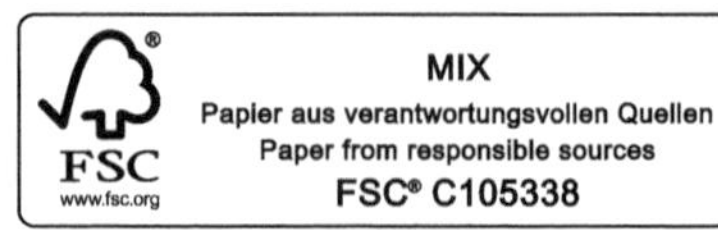

Printed by Books on Demand GmbH, Norderstedt / Germany